BETTER THAN EVER

The Fast-Track to Peak Performance in the Bedroom

Reclaiming your sex life <u>naturally</u>—regardless of age —without prescription drugs or surgery

John Byington with Robert W. Bly

Foreword by Leslie Cunningham, M.D.

Better Than Ever:
The Fast Track to Peak Performance In the Bedroom

Published by Agora Health Books

Alice Wessendorf, Managing editor
Ken Danz, Copy editor
Gerrit Wessendorf, Cover and book design

ISBN 1-891434-27-6

Printed in the United States of America

Agora Health Books
819 N. Charles Street
Baltimore, Maryland 21201
www.agorahealthbooks.com

Better Than Ever:
The Fast-Track to Peak Performance in the Bedroom

Reclaiming your sex life <u>naturally</u>—regardless of age
—without prescription drugs or surgery

John Byington with Robert W. Bly

Foreword by Leslie Cunningham, M.D.

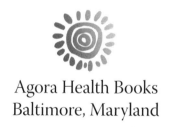

Agora Health Books
Baltimore, Maryland

DISCLAIMER

All material in this publication is provided for information only and may not be construed as medical advice or instruction. This book is intended as a reference only. The information given is designed to help make informed decisions about your health. No action should be taken based solely on the contents of this publication; instead, readers should consult appropriate health professionals on any matter relating to their health and well-being.

The authors of this book are not attempting to provide advice on the treatment or prevention of disease. Dietary supplements are not used to diagnose, prevent, or treat any disease. This book was not written to endorse the use of any products—natural or synthetic—for any treatment purpose or health benefit. The conclusions represent the authors' opinions of medical, scientific, folkloric, and lay writings on the various health care topics discussed.

The information and opinions provided in this book are believed to be accurate and sound, based on the best judgment available to the authors, but readers who fail to consult with appropriate health authorities assume the risk of any injuries.

The publishers and the authors accept no responsibility for the use of any agents mentioned in this book. Before an individual self-medicates, he or she is advised to seek the advice of a qualified health care professional.

TABLE OF CONTENTS

Chapter 1

Chapter 2

Chapter 3

Chapter 4

DEDICATION

For Eveline

—John Byington

For Amy

—Bob Bly

ACKNOWLEDGMENTS

Thanks to Dr. Leslie Cunningham, for her enthusiastic contributions to this project.

Thanks also to Dr. Seth Friedman, who contributed research and text.

Thanks to Gina Bilwin for her contributions in editing.

Thanks to Rachel Balcom for her research and editorial assistance.

Finally, thanks to our agent, Bob Diforio, for having faith in us and in this project.

FOREWORD

By Leslie Cunningham, M.D.

Children's Hospital of New Mexico,
Dept. of Pediatrics

When Viagra first came on the market, it was seen by many men over 40 as the perfect solution to their declining performance in the bedroom, the return of the rock-hard penis of their teenage years.

Not necessarily.

In this book, John Byington describes the drawbacks of the rock-hard erections produced by erectile dysfunction drugs and the holistic advantages of the natural alternatives.

For example, in a conversation with John and his wife Eveline, she told me that many menopausal women may find the "wooden penis" E.D. drugs create less than ideal. "What am I going to do with *that*?" many women wonder. "For me to become aroused, I need a lot of time for exploration and foreplay; quick intercourse is not what I'm after."

In the same chat, John emphasized to me the joys of broadening the boundaries of sexuality to include the realms of emotional and spiritual communication. Both John and Eveline believe that when quick sex becomes a problem, mature couples can choose to "become vulnerable and experimental in their sexual explorations."

Yes, such a path requires courage and a willingness to take new risks; people who are unwilling to take those risks may find their sex lives gradually disappearing. Read this book and discover what new sensations await you.

Preface

"Is sex dirty?
Only if it's done right."

—Woody Allen

According to recent surveys, one in ten males age 18 to 59 is unable to maintain an erection throughout sexual activity. Moreover, an article in the *Journal of Clinical Practice* reports that over half of men age 40 to 70 years old have some degree of "erection inadequacy."

Dr. Edward Moss, editor of *Urology and You*, estimates that there are more than 25 million impotent men in the United States. In 1985 the National Ambulatory Medical Care Survey reported that for every 1,000 men in the United States 7.7 visits to the doctors office were for erectile dysfunction. By 1999 that number nearly tripled to 22.3.

Why the sharp rise in the numbers of visits? The truth is there are probably a number of factors, not the least of which is the graying of the population. As the baby boom generation ages, according to some sources, approximately every 7 seconds another one of us turns 50. Since sexual potency naturally declines with age it is only to be expected that increasing numbers of us experience trouble having or maintaining erections. The fact is that the average 65-year-old, for example, has less than one-third the testosterone level of a normal 20-year-old man.

However there are other factors that can effect the quality and quantity of our sexual encounters. Stress, financial pressure, job responsibilities, parenting responsibilities, fatigue, illness, time, and other obligations often result in less opportunity for sex or less than satisfactory. In fact, three out of ten U.S. males surveyed say they have sex only a few times a year at most.

An increasing number of men have turned to prescription drugs to restore their potency. It is estimated that well over 1.5 million prescriptions for Viagra have been written since the drug's FDA approval in March 1998. Users of the high-profile drug have included Hugh Hefner and Bob Dole.

While Viagra was the first super-star erectile-dysfunction drug to hit the market it was soon followed by Cialis and Levitra in 2003. All three drugs are PDE5 inhibitors and they work by blocking a chemical in the penis that typically causes erections to subside.

The three drugs normally begin to work 30 to 45 minutes after taking them. Viagra and Levitra will typically stay in your system for about 4-6 hours. Cialis is usually effective for up to 24-36 hours after it is taken.

Viagra, Cialis, and Levitra have all become widely popular. With increasing numbers of men experiencing erectile dysfunction (E.D.) the subject has become much less of a taboo. It is not at all uncommon to see television commercials for E.D. drugs during prime time or during sports coverage (in fact Levitra is an official sponsor of the NFL). This openness around a previously "unmentionable" issue has undoubtedly had an impact on the numbers of men seeking out help from their doctors.

But sexual potency seekers and their physicians became more cautious about E.D. drugs after some of its possible side effects became widely publicized. Sobering headlines, like "16 Took Viagra and Died, FDA: No Link Yet, but Drug Eyed" that ran in New York *Daily News* quieted some of the enthusiasm over the drugs.

Adverse reactions in clinical tests of Viagra include headache, nasal congestion, urinary tract infection, diarrhea, dizziness, indigestion, edema, pain, chills, shock, migraine, rash, depression, and insomnia. Some who have taken the drug have suffered heart problems ranging from angina and abnormal electro-cardiograms, to palpitations and heart failure. In addition, one out of ten subjects in clinical trials experienced abnormal vision changes after taking 100 mg of Viagra daily.

Reported side effects of Cialis include headache, back pain, muscle pain, nasal congestion, flushing, limb pain, bowel complaints/indigestion. Less common, but perhaps more concerning, are the possible heart related side effects including angina, chest pain, hypotension, hypertension, heart attack, irregular heat beat and the digestive related side effects including abnormal liver function, gastro reflux, upper abdominal pain, diarrhea, and vomiting. Similar to Viagra, Cialis users may experience visual disturbances such as changes in color vision, blurred vision as well as eye pain and swelling of the eye lids.

Levitra like the other two E.D. drugs has a similar list of possible side-effects including headaches, flushing, nausea, heartburn, stuffy or runny, nose, and vision disturbances (blue auras around objects, an inability to distinguish between blue and green, blurred vision). In addition Levitra has possible heart related side effects as well including chest pain and irregular heart beat.

As dangerous as some of the side-effects of E.D. drugs may be, many men find surgery, implants, penile injections, vacuum therapy, and other alternatives even more daunting or distasteful. Research shows that while 95% of impotent men can be treated successfully, fewer than 5% have been treated.

The good news is: that many men can enjoy sexual potency equivalent to or better than what the E.D. drugs, provide without their harmful side effects, using natural alternatives. These include vitamins, minerals, herbs, amino acids, and other dietary supplements.

This is the strategy to enhance male sexual potency—safely and effectively—*Better than Ever: The Fast Track to Peak Performance In the Bedroom* will be focusing on.

The book presents a wealth of natural alternatives. Some have been a part of indigenous and folk medicine for centuries while others are more recently documented in clinical studies and professional medical journal articles. These alternatives have been known to offer benefits to men experiencing diminishing sex drive and performance including:

- a significant increase in the enjoyment of sex
- an easier time achieving an erection
- harder and longer-lasting erections
- more frequent and pleasurable sex
- enhanced ability to satisfy your partner
- more intense orgasms
- avoidance of prescription drugs' side effects
- more confidence in the bedroom
- money saved by avoiding fraudulent and ineffective cures

- eliminating premature ejaculation

- a noticeable improvement in sexual desire

- improved vitality, energy, and overall wellness.

Here's how this easy to follow guide is organized:

Chapter 1 covers the background and issues of male potency and sexual performance. Chapter 2 examines prescription E.D. drugs and other non-natural alternatives, exploring their positive effects as well as their dangers. These alternatives include penile injections, implants, devices, and microsurgery.

Chapters 3 provides an extensive consumer's guide to the natural male potency vitamins, herbs, and amino acids—including what they are, what they do, how they work, levels of effectiveness, recommended dosages and formulations, as well as side effects and appropriate warnings.

Chapter 4 examines other ways men can extend peak sexual potency into their middle and later years without costly prescription drugs or risky surgery.

Appendix A provides a directory of sources and resources from whom the reader can get additional information or order various supplements or supplies. Appendix B is a glossary.

In Search of an Orgasm:
Mature Male Sexuality...
a State of the Union Address

*"There may be some things better
than sex, and some things may
be worse. But there is nothing
exactly like it."*

—W.C. Fields

This is a true story. It happened only a couple of years ago. After twenty-five minutes of the best lovemaking we'd had in months, my wife Eveline leaned back on the pillow, her eyes closed, a faint blush on her bare chest.

Slowly, she opened her eyes and, smiling, looked at me admiringly.

"Wow," she said. "John, what happened? I mean, we both know sex hasn't been—well—the best lately..."

"Let's be honest," I laughed. "It's been virtually nonexistent...and we both know the reason."

She ran her hand down my chest, onto my stomach, slowly toward my groin, where I felt a stirring I hadn't felt for a long time, until a few months ago.

"So what happened just now?" she asked with excitement in her voice. "Sex was great—just like when we were first dating!"

Although she and I are middle-aged, she's still gorgeous. *Still beautiful*, I thought as we relaxed in our bed.

"Well, I suppose you could mostly thank Dr. Friedman for tonight," I began.

She sat up, concerned. Dr. Friedman was my prostate specialist, and I had had prostate cancer several years ago—part of the reason, we knew, for my fading sex drive and problems maintaining an erection.

"John," she asked in a worried voice, her eyes wide with concern. "Is something wrong?"

"Relax," I said, hugging her to reassure her. "Nothing's wrong, and my cancer hasn't come back. In fact," I said, looking down the length of the blanket, "things are better there than ever before—and they're going to stay that way."

"How?" Eveline asked, genuinely curious.

This is the story I told her and now want to share with you….

The Viagra Generation

Millions of men today don't have the sex life, sex drive, or sexual potency they wish they did. Many are headed in the direction of totally giving up sex. *But you and I don't have to.*

How do I know?

I know because, as former director of Southwest Research Institute—a cooperative of doctors and scientists doing leading-edge research in male sexual potency—one of my most rewarding tasks was talking to men all over the U.S. These men, ages 40 to 80+, were remarkably frank about their desire to amplify and intensify their sexual experiences.

It wasn't uncommon to hear comments like, "I've been impotent", "I can't get it up. Makes me feel awful", "Makes me feel like less of a man", "My wife is understanding, but you know I used to be able to get it up all the time", or "I can't get it up. What's going on?" It's not that they cried then, but they may have *felt* like crying. That's the vulnerability. They talked about their illnesses too. Guys over 45 and 50, parts of us start to break down, and when we break down we become vulnerable—unless we are some kind of macho creature, which is not very enjoyable to be around or to talk to.

I listened to the men who said, "I've been sick, I hurt, my joints hurt, you know, and my prostrate gland doesn't work." Or, "I can't get it up the way I used to." That immediately evokes vulnerability.

These men were sincere and straightforward. As we talked, there was usually acknowledgment that we are aging, and don't have the hormonal input or overall health and vitality we once had. Life takes a toll. But the one thing we have in common is: We all want to continue being men...and that includes having sex...for as long as we can.

According to a study conducted by Luntz Research for *Playboy* magazine, men—despite performance problems—feel they should be in control in bed. Six out of ten men surveyed say they almost always "take charge" during sex, and half say they are "more adventuresome in bed" than their female partners. At the same time, six out of ten say it is more difficult to be a man today than it was twenty years ago.

If you are frustrated by a declining sex life, be comforted in knowing you're not alone. Far from it. As Eric Yudelove observes in his book *100 Days to Better Health, Good Sex & Long Life* (Llewellyn Press), "For men over 40, the emphasis of lovemaking shifts away from the quick orgasm toward sustained ability to maintain an erection."

Here are the facts: In a Gallup Poll taken for the American Medical Association 12% of the men interviewed said they had experienced sexual difficulty related to impotence. While 65% of the men and women interviewed said they had sexual intercourse in the past month, that figure dropped to 28% for men and women over 65.

Meanwhile, a study sponsored by the John D. and Catherine T. MacArthur Foundation found that men and women ages 40 to 60 rated their sex lives only 5.5 on a scale of 1 to 10. According to an article in the *Journal of the American Medical Association (JAMA)*, 33% of 1,410 men between ages 18 and 59 said they had a persistent problem of climaxing early. And 14% said they had no interest in sex.

It is reported that 52% of men between ages 40 and 70 suffer from some degree of erectile dysfunction, and more than 25 million men are going through "male menopause." Male menopause is a somewhat controversial stage, which supposedly involves hormonal shifts that can affect mood, physical well-being, and sexuality; symptoms include reduced libido, fear of sexual failure, fatigue, and sleep disturbances.

Writing in *Longevity Quarterly* (Vol. 5, No. 1, page 9), Dr. Larry Doss observes that nearly one out of five men age 55 report potency difficulties. That number jumps to more than one in two men by age 75. The inability to achieve an erection, *impotence*, affects almost 10 million American men.

If you once could do the deed but now cannot, are you impotent? According to William Masters and Virginia Johnson, in their book *Human Sexual Inadequacy* (Little, Brown and Company), "When an individual male's rate of failure at successful coital connection approaches 25% of his opportunities, the clinical diagnosis of … impotence must be accepted." In other words, if one out of four times that you attempt sex you are unable to complete the act then you suffer from impotence.

The inability to get or maintain an erection can occur at any time during a man's life and for a wide variety of reasons. If your impotence does not have a physiological cause you most likely continue to have erections while you sleep. Urologists use special devices to measure your "nocturnal penile tumescence" but a simple at home test can help you determine whether you are still getting erections while you sleep. Simply wrap a coil of postage stamps around your penis before going to sleep. In the morning if the stamps are torn you probably experienced a normal erection during your sleep.

What Causes Impotence?

Dr. Edward Moss, a urologist, includes among the main causes of impotence arterial sclerosis (hardening of the arteries), diabetes, Alzheimer's disease, Parkinson's disease, Multiple Sclerosis, trauma, paralysis, stroke, thyroid and pituitary problems, loss of testosterone, and certain forms of surgery and radiation therapy. Other frequent causes of impotence are stress, depression, boredom, side effects from prescription medications (especially blood pressure drugs), smoking, alcohol, and—not to be ignored—performance anxiety.

Additional causes of impotence can include vascular disease, heart disease, neurologic impairment, psychological disorders, pelvic injury, hormonal imbalance, peyronie's disease (a rare condition that can cause inflammation and bending of the penis) and smoking. According to the journal *Urology*, smoking is the biggest contributing factor in impotence; one study found that in a group of 1,000 men suffering from impotence, almost four out of five were smokers.

TABLE 1

PHYSICAL CAUSES OF IMPOTENCE

Anatomic

- Congenital deformities
- Testicular fibrosis
- Hydrocele

Cardiorespiratory

- Angina pectoris
- Myocardial infarction
- Emphysema
- Rheumatic fever
- Coronary insufficiency
- Pulmonary insufficiency

Drug Ingestion

- Addictive drugs
- Alcohol
- Alph-methyl-dopa
- Amphetamines
- Atropine
- Chlordiazepoxide
- Chlorprothixene
- Guanethidine
- Imipramine
- Methantheline bromide
- Monoamine oxidase inhibitors
- Phenothiazines
- Reserpine
- Thioridazine
- Nicotine
- Digitalis

Endocrine

- Acromegaly
- Addison's disease
- Adrenal neoplasmas (with or without Cushing's syndrome)
- Castration
- Chromophobe adenoma
- Craniopharyngioma
- Diabetes mellitus
- Eunuchoidism (including Klinefelter's syndrome
- Feminizing interstitial-cell testicular tumors
- Infantilism
- Ingestion of female hormones (estrogen)
- Myxedema
- Obesity
- Thyrotoxicosis

Genitourinary

- Perineal prostatectomy
- Prostatitis
- Phimosis
- Priapism
- Suprapubic and transurethral prostatectomy
- Urethritis

Hematologic

- Hodgkin's disease
- Leukemia, acute and chronic
- Primary anemia

Infectious

- Genital tuberculosis
- Gonorrhea
- Mumps

Neurologic

- Amyotrophic lateral sclerosis
- Cord tumors or transection
- Electric shock therapy
- Multiple sclerosis
- Nutritional deficiencies
- Parkinsonism
- Peripheral neuropathies
- Spina bifida
- Sympathectomy
- Tabes dorsalis
- Temporal lobe lesions

Vascular

- Aneurysm
- Arteritis
- Sclerosis
- Thrombotic obstruction of aortic bifurcation

Source: *Human Sexual Inadequacy* (Little, Brown and Company)

Dr. Edwin Flatto, in his book *Super Potency at Any Age* (Instant Improvement), says that in one British study, half the diabetic men examined complained of impotence. Other causes of impotence listed by Dr. Flatto include high blood pressure, liver or kidney failure, fractures in the pelvic area, spinal cord injuries, congenital hormonal problems, sickle-cell anemia, hyper and hypo-thyroidism, aortic aneurysm surgery, lead poisoning, Leriche's syndrome, and Lou Gehrig's disease.

> **S**moking increases the risk of erectile dysfunction by up to 50% for men in their 30s and 40s.

According to Flatto, booze, not cigarettes, is the number one substance abuse problem leading to male sexual dysfunction. He says that four out of five men who drink heavily are believed to suffer from impotence, sterility, loss of sexual desire, and other sexual problems.

Many prescription medicines, especially those for circulatory conditions and depression, can contribute to male sexual dysfunction. An article posted on MedicineNet.com says side effects from drugs—both prescription and illegal—account for one out of four cases of impotence.

According to *Intimacy & Depression: The Silent Epidemic*, a booklet published by Glaxo Wellcome, antidepressants may interfere with sexual drive, arousal, function, satisfaction, and orgasm. "It can be difficult to differentiate the sexual disinterest so common in depression from the sexual disinterest seen with some antidepressant medications." Their recommendation: Communicate your reactions to medication to your doctor and ask his or her advice.

It is estimated that up to 140 million men suffer from impotence worldwide. In addition, 350,000 men annually in the United States have prostate problems—and many suffer a diminished sex life as a result. In fact, 60% of men ages 40 to 59 suffer from enlargement of the prostate, called benign prostate hyperplasia (BPH).

I was one of those men. And frankly, I didn't like what was happening to me. I was preoccupied with my pelvic area, and I was letting it run my whole life.

I'd feel tired, and the next thing I knew, I started to give up on an area of my life that had been important to me for many, many years: an active sex life. I was reminded of what playwright Henry Miller said about making love: "Sex is one of the nine reasons for reincarnation … and the other eight are unimportant."

With me having suffered from both colon and prostate cancer, Eveline and I have been through some very rough times.

She's one of the two most important people who helped me get through my health crisis. The other is my physician, Dr. Seth Friedman, who treated my prostate cancer.

While I was in treatment, Seth and I became good friends. Our friendship has continued ever since. It led me to embark on a journey into alternative medical treatments for sexual dysfunction that most men have not explored. But for those of you who do, it can be a new avenue of hope—and a road back to the vigorous sex life you enjoyed years ago, in your teens and twenties. This sounds almost too good to be true, I know. But this book—your clear guide to these natural alternatives—will give you the facts.

Think of your penis as a messenger. If things are not right in your life either psychologically or physically your penis is going to let you know. Your erections can be effected by everything from stress, to exhaustion, to diet. And remember impotence can be an early warning sign of arterial problems such as an impending hear attack or stroke so be sure to check with your doctor if you suddenly are experiencing problems.

The most important fact is: You *can* restore and enhance your sexual performance—without taking prescription drugs. You *can* get and sustain frequent, hard, long-lasting erections…without vacuum pumps, rings, implants, or surgery.

In this book, you'll discover:

- Why you're not alone…and why so many men see their sex lives slipping away as the years go by.

- The truth about prescription drugs and other "cures" prescribed by the medical establishment.

- How to restore your sexual potency and sex drive through safe, effective, natural alternatives to prescription drugs—including foods, herbs, vitamins, amino acids, and other supplements… most of which you can buy at the health food store, pharmacy, or even your neighborhood supermarket.

- How to manage your newly invigorated sexual functionality so that it strengthens—rather than weakens—the physical and emotional bonds between you and your partner.

- What you can do in your lifestyle—health, diet, exercise, and in the bedroom—to maximize your sexual health, performance, and pleasure for a lifetime.

Why Sexual Ability Changes With Age

Sex is central to our culture. For instance, a Kaiser Foundation study of more than 1,300 TV shows found that 56% of these programs had some depiction of sexual activities, which researchers defined as flirting, passionate kissing, talking about sex, and intercourse. Sex is depicted in eight out of ten soap operas, 83% of TV movies, and is discussed on three out of four talk shows.

Aging is almost as great a fear in our culture as sexual inadequacy. Your sex life at 20, 40, 50, or 60 doesn't need to be exactly the same. It's very likely that your views of sex, and what's really important in a partner, will change through time. After all, most of our views evolve as we mature.

Every man has the experience of growing older and having sexual virility wane. Tables 2-3 tell the story. At age 15, the body's testosterone levels and overall health can lead to repeated erections and a very short refractory time (the time it takes to regain an erection after orgasm). Once we hit age 40, our testosterone level decreases about 1% a year from then on.

With a reputed peak of virility at 18, the myth is that sex is all downhill after that. It is true that a man's ability to get and sustain erections may lessen as he ages. It may take longer to regain an erection, or you may manage only one erection. Erections themselves may be soft or non-existent. It's also true that a key organ of male sexuality, the prostate, begins slowly growing after age 40 and can lead to various problems. The trend throughout a man's life is clear. The question is, "What can be done about it?"

Men actually have two different types of erections. The first is a reflexogenic erection, which is the kind you get from direct stimulation of your genitals. The second type of erections, psychogenic erections, are the kind that are stimulated by something we see, think about, or even smell. So for example seeing a pretty girl in a skirt walk by might trigger a psychogenic erection. Or later fantasizing about that girl or smelling the same perfume she was wearing might bring on a psychogenic erection.

As a natural progression of aging we start to lose our psychogenic erections. The problem is nobody bothers to tell us about this. Women are prepared to start experiencing certain changes as they age such as vaginal dryness and hot flashes as their hormones change, but men are never taught that they too should expect changes as they age as well. So instead of realizing that this psychogenic erection response naturally dulls as we age we start to think we can't get erections like we used to and we assume we are impotent. The next step is avoiding sex and eventually starting to lose the urge altogether.

TABLE 2

Male potency as a function of age

Potency Facts	Age 20	Age 30	Age 40	Age 50	Age 60	Age 70
Incidence of Impotence			5%		15-33%	3%
Zero to Tumescence (Erection) (Avg. in seconds)		3-5		6-10		9-30
Avg. Angle of Erection (Degrees above (+) or below (-) Horizontal)	20+	0+	0-		25-	
Testosterone in Normal Body (Avg. nanograms/L)	175	150	125		55 (at age 65)	
Average Annual Orgasms (Total)	104	121	84	52	35	22
Rest Required Between Orgasms	minutes		up to hours		many hours	

First, a man's sexual appetite and ability will carry through from his youth. "Relative frequency of sexual activity does not change with age," writes Leonard Hayflick in his book *How and Why We Age* (Ballantine). "The men who were most sexually active in their 70s were also highly active sexually in their 20s." That's the baseline, one might say.

Different men start adult life with different appetites. Having reasonable expectations dictates that we accept our own sexual nature rather than compare it with the locker-room tales of our friends. If we didn't have the same appetites and attitudes as our peers at 18, we'll march to a different drummer at 28, at 38, and at 88.

Secondly, the rate of change in a man's sexuality can differ. It's this rate that we have some control over. By taking a more mature perspective in understanding male sexuality, we can often sustain our sexual health over a lifetime. The abilities of a teenager aren't the abilities of an adult male. The skills and enthusiasms of an adult male aren't those of a teenager.

Changes in lifestyle, diet and behavior can help maintain good physical health and thereby sustain good sexual health. Something as simple as yoga, tai chi or stretching exercises can often lead to a newfound level of flexibility and relaxation in the body. Men, at any age, can learn something new and enjoyable about how their body works. They can tune their body to work well, with or without a partner. The goal is a sex life that sustains and nourishes you at every stage of life. Chapter 4 gives you specific how-to instructions on things you can do in diet and exercise to enhance your sex life well into your later years.

Menopause, His and Hers

Sexual expression takes place in a partnership. Anxiety is the greatest killer of sexual happiness. It's important to put yourself in a sexual situation where anxiety is minimized and where sexual satisfaction is most likely. A partner's transition through menopause can mean months or several years of transition, and a man is part of that change. Some medical practitioners actually believe that there is a similar change of life for men, called male menopause or "andropause." It's still being debated.

Most men, somewhere between the age of 40 and 60, pause and begin to reflect about their lives and their futures. Just as you have to adapt to your partner's experiences, your partner needs to take your views into account. The trust necessary to talk about what you want is often the same trust your partner seeks.

Mutually satisfying sex can make a good marriage better. According to research compiled by the National Council on Aging, more than 70% of sexually active older people say that sex is as emotionally satisfying as when they were in their 40s. "Sexuality remains a vital element in the lives of older people," says James P. Firman, president of the council.

Dissatisfaction in your love life can be a vicious cycle leading to stress and further dissatisfaction. Playfulness in the bedroom is an excellent remedy for breaking that cycle. Sex should be fun and recreational. And remember a sense of humor is an essential ingredient in a good sex life. It takes the pressure off and allows you both to release all kinds of feel-good hormones.

Men and women are unique in the animal kingdom. Most mammals are naturally bound to restrict their sexual activity to well-defined cycles when climate and availability of food and water are advantageous for breeding. This is of course not true for humans. Freed from the bridle of outside rhythms "that which distinguishes man from beast is drinking without being thirsty and making love at all seasons" (from *The Marriage of Figaro*). That's why we wrote this book. We offer it to men in all seasons of life to support, inspire and inform you so that your physical and sexual energy can be completely available to you, giving you and your partner

TABLE 3

Frequency of sex as a function of age

Frequency of Sex in the Past Twelve Months by Age, Marital Status, and Gender

Social characteristics	Not at all	A few times per year	A few times per month	2 or 3 times a week	4 or more times a week
GENDER					
Men	14%	16%	37%	26%	8%
Women	10	18	36	30	7
AGE					
Men					
18-24	15	21	24	28	12
25-29	7	15	31	36	11
30-39	8	15	37	33	6
40-49	9	18	40	27	6
50-59	11	22	43	20	3
Women					
18-24	11	16	32	29	12
25-29	5	10	38	37	10
30-39	9	16	36	33	6
40-49	15	16	44	20	5
50-59	30	22	35	12	2
MARITAL/RESIDENTIAL STATUS					
Men					
Noncohabiting	23	25	26	19	7
Cohabiting	0	8	36	40	16
Married	1	13	43	36	7
Women					
Noncohabiting	32	23	24	15	5
Cohabiting	1	8	35	42	14
Married	3	12	47	32	7

Source: *Sex in America*

physical intimacy that is more satisfying, scintillating and alive.

Sex is a central and undeniable part of any man's life. But given the changeable, high-stress atmosphere most of us live in today, having a contented sex life can seem like an unattainable goal for a man. Typically, men aren't apt to think or talk much about their bodies—at least not anything north of their thigh muscles or south of their pecs. The average guy knows a lot more about his car than he does about his own body. Whatever has caused men to avoid learning, they are generally hesitant to talk openly or seriously about physical health, the bad habits that may be affecting it, and what's going on inside the outer husk.

Partly, this is due to a lack of awareness. Partly, it is anxiety. And part of it may be the way our culture has taught us to behave. We want to have and give the impression of being in control of our lives, to the envy of some and the suspicion of others. Underneath we feel semi-powerless to affect the direction of our work, our relationships, and even what happens in sex. We joke about growing old. We alternately joke or boast about our virility. Underneath the jokes, we worry and make silent confessions.

What Makes for a Good Lover?

A good lover is someone who goes beyond "what comes naturally" to learn and practice ways of generating partnership and pleasure for himself and those with whom he shares his bed. Men today have become newly interested in discussing and actively cultivating their sexual skills by applying techniques and nutritional support from both ancient and modern sources, to give themselves and their partners greater sexual pleasure.

Keeping pace with the women of today and modern life, we must change with the times. Many men, by themselves or in groups, are starting to question the values with which they were raised. Questioning what those values mean today and what price they exact, they are also re-evaluating what it means to be a man, what kind of man they want to be, and how they can maintain sexual vigor in the face of it all.

Is your sex life a chore or a blessing? Do you face the coming years confident and relaxed? Or are you worried that your partner won't find you as attractive and sexually skilled as you once were?

In our society, with its bias toward youth, older men who are still interested in sex are sometimes considered with amusement, curiosity, disdain, or (perhaps secretly) envy. But if we listen to the ancient Taoist masters from China and the wisdom of other cultures, sex is revered as a lifelong activity that is possible and desirable until the day we die.

Many men report that their sex life improved after making a commitment to a partner or tying the knot. To assure you are one of these committed <u>and</u> happy guys think variety. And while novelty is good for your sex life you don't necessarily mean have to take a walk on the wild side. Just changing routines or locations can give the added spark you are looking for.

No two men are alike. They certainly aren't alike when it comes to their sexual health, desires and expectations. But there are some common experiences which men can share to grant us more scintillating sex that is part of our birthright.

The Best Sex You Ever Had

If you think back to the sexual experiences that were the most deeply satisfying for you, chances are you were in a place, mood or physical condition that was particularly positive. Feeling good—mentally and physically—makes it more likely that we will have good sexual experiences: Our bodies require a certain degree of well-being, overall security, and acceptance before we can have genuine interest and energy for lovemaking.

Whatever your personal precondition for good sex is, it's yours. There is no standard or common ground that defines or judges one man's sex life versus another's. And we certainly can't compare what happens for us between the sheets with anything we read or see in the entertainment media. What's yours is yours. However, we can look at some basic physiological factors that optimize the body's readiness and willingness to be sexual and satisfy those basic needs.

To fully express male sexual health, you need:

- Adequate health—taking care of your physical and emotional well-being.

- Knowledge—having a basic understanding of your body's sexual organs and systems.

- Reasonable expectations—understanding what you can reasonably expect from your body.

- Awareness and instruction in energy-generating techniques— using your breath, muscles, and imagination to create more scintillating experiences.

Together these elements can make a world of difference in the quality and quantity of your sex life. They can enhance your life with esteem and continued sexual success, which can make a big contribution to your overall happiness and vitality.

Reviewing Man's Body: What's Under the Hood?

The human, mammalian body that you have is the crowning product of a long evolution. There are some basic facts about it that you might want to get familiar with, though there's no need to obsess about them. You just might want to know what you have that's really unique. Knowing the "basics" not only helps you understand your body; it can also enhance your own sexual health and contentment.

To begin with, we can plainly see that our sexual apparatus is on the outside. The penis and testicles are familiar sex organs...and pretty much the main ones we identify with. To understand male sexual functioning more thoroughly, though, let's start by looking inside (Figure. 1).

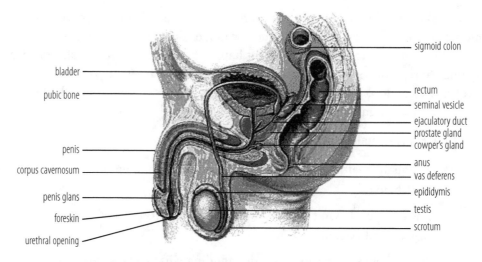

sigmoid colon

bladder

pubic bone

rectum
seminal vesicle
ejaculatory duct
prostate gland
cowper's gland

penis

corpus cavernosum

anus
vas deferens

penis glans

epididymis

foreskin

testis

urethral opening

scrotum

Figure 1: Drawing of the Male Internal Sexual Anatomy

First, notice the scrotum, the fleshy pouch that houses our testicles, where sperm is created and stored. By being located on the exterior of our body, the pouch manages to keep the temperature cool enough for sperm to survive. That's why wearing briefs—tight underwear which holds the testicles against the warm body—instead of loose boxers is often discouraged for men who are trying to conceive a baby and may be suffering from low sperm count or motility. There is some question about whether or not this is at all effective. But it certainly can't hurt.

From the testicles, a set of tubes called the *vas deferens* carry the sperm on its journey from each testicle up into the interior of the body. These two vas tubes then connect to a walnut-sized gland called the prostate. The prostate and the two nearby seminal vesicles together create a fluid base for the sperm, called semen. It's the seminal fluid that we see during ejaculation.

The seminal fluid contains various proteins, chemicals, and fructose, which serve as nutrients for the sperm cells. Each milliliter of semen (a milliliter is less than half an eye-dropper full) contains about 100 million sperm.

A normal human cell has forty-six chromosomes, but a sperm cell

---

Testicular Self-Exam

If you are not doing a testicular self-exam once a month you should be. It's important to become familiar with how your testicles feel when they are healthy so you can easily recognize if something is different.

The best place to do the check is in the bath or shower when the skin of the scrotum will be most relaxed.

Hold the scrotum in the palms of your hands and use your fingers and thumbs to feel your testicles. It is normal to have differences between the two testicles like one being larger than the other or hanging lower. Gently roll the testicles between your thumb and forefinger and then gently press each one.

At the top and back of both testicles you will find there is a soft tube. This tube is the epididymis, which stores and carries sperm. Running up from the epididymis is a smooth tube.

Check for any small irregularities, enlargements, or changes in firmness. Both testicles should be smooth with no lumps or swellings. Often there is no pain associated with a lump, but you may find there is a dull ache. Since it is rare to develop cancer in both testicles at once if you feel something that worries you compare the questionable testicle with the other.

No matter how small, a lump should be taken seriously. If you find a lump, swelling, or change in your testicles go see your doctor. However, don't panic! Keep in mind that most lumps or swellings found in the in the testicles are not cancer but rather benign cysts or fatty tissue. It's still important to get them checked out to rule out any problems and to put your mind at ease.

---

has only twenty-three—half the usual number. When it combines with the twenty-three chromosomes in the female egg, the human thus conceived has the full complement of forty-six chromosomes.

You've probably seen pictures of the sperm depicting it as an oval head with a long tail. The tail is made of protein fibers that contract on alternate sides, creating a wave-like movement that propels the sperm through the seminal fluid and toward the egg.

The prostate sits just under the bladder—a sponge-like organ where urine collects in the body before it is expelled. Another tube, called the urethra, starts at the bladder, and passes through the prostate on its way out of the body via the penis.

The tube of the urethra passes urine all the way to the head of the penis.

The prostate could be considered a switching station within the male sexual system. A series of muscles and muscular valves control whether semen or urine will pass through the urethra, depending on what activity this part of your body is engaged in. All of this happens pretty much automatically and is not something we voluntarily control. (You've probably noticed you often need to urinate not long after an ejaculation. This is the body's way of clearing the urethra of leftover sperm so that the tube remains unblocked.)

When a man gets stimulated sexually, something called nitric oxide (NO) is produced and released in the large blood vessels of the penis. NO helps to create and maintain erections. Blood vessels in the penis open wide to allow blood to enter and engorge the area expanding the spongy tissue of the penis known as the corpus cavernosum.

As this expansion occurs, the veins at the base of the penis, which would normally allow blood to leave, get compressed. Since the veins are pinched off, our blood gets trapped in the shaft of the penis, causing the hardness we know and love. The erection continues as long as there is stimulation, causing more nitric oxide production to keep the erectile tissue hard from the inflow of blood that can't exit.

DID YOU KNOW?

Men ejaculate at an average speed of 28 miles per hour!

While all this is going on, signals from the nervous system promote movement of the sperm-rich seminal fluid in anticipation of ejaculation. Internal valves at the root of the penis, near the prostate, divert the flow and direction within the urethra to prepare for the passage of semen.

At climax, the man ejaculates, expelling semen from the tip of the penis. After ejaculation, the veins open again, allowing the blood to re-enter normal circulation, where it is reoxygenated by the heart and lungs. The penis relaxes and softens from the outflow of blood, and our bodies enter a recovery period while sperm-count rises again. The body is simultaneously able to produce more nitric oxide, so that erection is again possible.

Orgasm is initiated in this way at the gonads, traveling from the rhythmic contraction of muscles in the groin and engaging all aspects of the nervous system. The mechanics of ejaculation may or may not be accompanied by orgasm, in which the whole body enters a state of heightened sensations, receptivity, relaxation, and then rest.

Pioneering sex researchers William Masters and Virginia Johnson describe orgasm as "sudden, rhythmic muscular contractions in the pelvic region and elsewhere in the body that releases accumulated sexual tension and the mental sensations accompanying that experience." They distinguish it from ejaculation, which is simply a reflex that occurs at the base of the spine to release semen.

The Reichian school of psychotherapy makes a distinction between *climax*, as the muscular contractions in the genitals, and *orgasm*, which is described as contractions that spread throughout the entire body. On the continuum of sexual pleasure, the line between climax and orgasm is often blurry and varies at different times and also for each individual. So whatever you feel and whatever you want to call it, enjoy it!

Some orgasms are an explosive, ecstatic avalanche of sensations, while others are milder, less intense and dramatic. Biologically, orgasm is the shortest phase in the sexual response cycle, often lasting for only a few seconds. During these seconds, rhythmic muscular contractions produce intense physical sensation and skin flushing, followed by rapid relaxation.

Psychologically, orgasm is usually a time of suspended thought and extreme pleasure—the mind turns inward to enjoy the personal experience. Brain wave patterns show distinct changes during orgasm with differing intensities of response arising throughout the body. These are influenced by many factors such as fatigue, the time of the last orgasm, mood, your relationship with your partner, health, activity, sex-differences and expectations.

The Proof Is in Your Pants

Erection, ejaculation, and orgasm are how your body is meant to respond as a sexual being. Obviously though, we live in an imperfect world and things don't always work exactly according to plan. In fact, our bodies may seem to manifest weird symptoms or conditions at times.

The body naturally self-cleanses and restores positive balance and health. Even disease is an expression of the body's effort toward self-cure when overwhelmed by stressors that exceed its ability to adapt. What can lead to chronic disease are mistaken efforts to cure or suppress the body's efforts to cleanse, harmonize, and adapt itself. Downgraded health and disease can be eliminated by removing the real cause and by raising the body's general vitality. These two factors then allow our natural and innate ability of sustained health to dominate.

Men's bodies can handle tremendous amounts of stress and changes, but there are limits…and often the overwhelming nature of life is expressed in less than satisfying sex. Let's look at some of the problems that can occur in a man's body over time from genetic, environmental, nutritional, physical, or just unknown causes.

The Geezer Effect

Aging creates distinct physiological changes. Sometimes starting as early as in our 30's and 40's, men have to work a little harder to keep up their sexual vitality. The body's glands operate more sluggishly and produce lesser amounts of the hormones related to sexual activity. Some men notice longer gaps after orgasm before they begin to feel sexually motivated or "in the mood" again. This makes sense, as their bodies may take more time to rebuild the hormonal stores that sharpen male perceptions and behaviors. Problems like premature ejaculation or impotence, even if temporary, are not uncommon.

What can cause our sex drive to falter? Factors like poor nutrition, exposure to excessive stress, drugs and other toxins, circulatory problems, chronic disease, poor sleep and/or exercise habits can all pave the way to lower than expected deliveries and gratification in the sexual department. Too much alcohol can increase desire but impair your ability to perform; one study of 14,000 alcoholics over a 37-year period showed that almost one in ten suffered from total impotence.

Injury and disease can affect sexuality too. If blood circulation is impaired in some way, erectile function is affected. Blood then flows less briskly to the genitals, decreasing a man's ability to get and maintain hardness as desired. The end result for some is loss of sexual appetite or ability.

> *TIPS*
>
> Three quick tips for improving sexual function
>
> ❶ Exercise more
> ❷ Quit smoking
> ❸ Limit alcohol

Potency problems are reported to affect 50% of men occasionally and 13% of men constantly. If you find yourself sagging when you want to be wagging, you are not alone. A large percentage of cases have a physical cause. Arteriosclerosis (hardening of the arteries) and the drugs used to control blood pressure are two major contributors to erection problems. Remember, if it's good for your arteries it's also good for your penis. A visit to an internist or urologist is the first step to identifying such causes.

Stress is another major culprit in reducing sexual desire and ability. This means factors like lifestyle, eating habits, emotional difficulties, or even chemical exposure can poorly influence your interest and performance. The use of tobacco, alcohol, and recreational drugs that are often a part of modern sexual activity can actually dampen sexual vigor. There is also evidence that coffee and red wine can irritate the urinary tract and aggravate a tendency toward infection. Repeated use of alcohol can lower testosterone levels and have a significant impact on potency. Smoking has been associated with non-rigid erections, impotence, and overall lowered sperm counts, while coffee depletes the body of the mineral calcium—an important factor in nerve and muscle functioning.

High blood pressure can lead to a blockage of your arteries known as arteriosclerosis. This arteriosclerosis can block the arteries to the penis a leading cause of impotence. Be sure to get your blood pressure checked at least once a year. To lower borderline high blood pressure, after checking with your doctor, try exercising and a sensible weigh loss plan to bring those numbers down.

Did your erectile difficulties begin soon after starting a new drug? If so make sure to discuss this fact with your doctor. It's possible that the medication might be contributing to your problem. Common prescription medications such as blood pressure pills, antidepressants, sedatives, ulcer medications, hormones, and even some over the counter cold medicines can contribute to erectile problems. While the vast majority of men on these drugs will not experience impotence you should review your medications with your doctor if you are experiencing trouble.

Diseases can obviously affect not only our ability to perform sex but our desire for sex as well. Drug use, whether of prescription, non-prescription or illegal varieties, can also have a wide range of negative effects on sexual health. Numerous prescription medicines are known to cause occasional impotence; it's worth checking for listed side effects.

Low-level sleep deprivation has become widespread in industrialized, urban areas, and there are suspicions that it is having a long-term impact on health. And to top it all off, scientists have been discovering a worldwide drop in the sperm count of the average man. Certain herbs and vitamin-based supplements can be a gentle way of restoring the body's ability to let go into sleep and deeper relaxation, in turn allowing the body's reserves and systems to recharge themselves.

While some of the factors mentioned here are somewhat in our immediate control, several categories of health problems can affect the structural parts of your reproductive tract as well as how it functions. They are worth turning our attention to, since they can pose a threat to our health … and also put a damper on scintillating sex, should they happen to you.

Urethritis and Prostatitis

Urethritis is an infection of the urethra, the tube inside the penis. Prostatitis is an infection of the prostate. Typical symptoms of both are discomfort and pain, frequent urination, and sometimes blood in the urine. These infections can be either acute (short-term) or chronic (recurring). Such symptoms clearly detract from one's sexual health and sex life. Your physician can usually treat them effectively with antibiotics and other therapies. Urinary tract infections can also affect this area, making it difficult for urine to clear from the bladder. Medicine (both mainstream and alternative) can provide useful drugs, herbs and foods to help prevent or alleviate such infections.

The Aging Male Body

Let's face it guys as we get older physical changes to our bodies are inevitable. If we know what to expect when it comes to our own plumbing then we are less likely to be freaked out by these changes and to assume that there is something wrong. Following are some of the most common sexual changes you should expect as you get older.

- It may take longer for you to get an erection or more stimulation may be needed. In addition, the time it take to have another erection after orgasm (what is technically called the refractory period) increases and for some guys it may take up to 24 or even 48 hours.

- Your erections will most likely be less firm than in your younger days.

- Ejaculation will become less forceful and the actual volume of ejaculate normally decreases as a result of changes in your prostate.

- Orgasms may not always be accompanied with ejaculation since your prostate is not producing as much semen as it did before.

- You may experience more lost erections before having an orgasm than you did in your younger days.

- A bonus to aging, for both you and your partner, is that you most likely will be able to delay ejaculation for a longer period of time since you will often require more stimulation before ejaculation.

Benign Prostatic Hyperplasia: BPH

The prostate is a walnut-sized gland that forms part of the male reproductive system. The gland is made of two lobes, or regions, enclosed by an outer layer of tissue. As the diagrams in Figure 2 show, the prostate is located in front of the rectum and just below the bladder, where urine is stored. The prostate also surrounds the urethra, the canal through which urine passes out of the body. With BPH the prostate swells placing pressure on the urethra.

Figure 2: Normal Urine Flow and Urine Flow with BPH

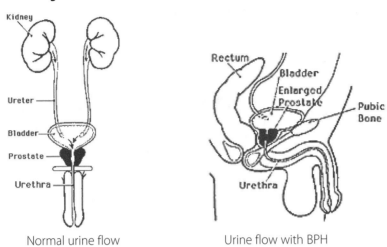

Normal urine flow   Urine flow with BPH

After the age of 40, the prostate can begin to swell in the *perineum*—the space between the scrotum and anus. This "hyperplasia" (overgrowth) is present in 50% of men aged 51-60 and continues to show up in a larger percentage of men as they age. As the word "benign" suggests, the problem isn't really a problem until the prostate's growth places pressure on the urethra passing through it, or the glands located within. Symptoms can include difficult or more frequent urination, or irritation in the urethra.

Approximately 350,000 men in the United States undergo surgery each year to clear obstructions of the urethra. Surgical intervention in advanced cases can have an impact on potency. Fortunately, there is a renaissance of natural (and pharmaceutical) substances receiving widespread attention for their potential to improve prostate health and prevent BPH before it becomes problematic. Saw palmetto and pygeum africanum (covered in Chapter 3) are key among the natural remedies. New, less invasive surgical techniques have also been developed to correct BPH with less disruption of a man's sex life.

Prostate Cancer

Prostate carcinoma is the second most prominent cancer in North American men, outstripped only by skin cancer. It is second only to lung cancer in the number of men's lives it takes. Rates have been on the rise. Age, genetic inheritance, and male hormones have a role in prostate carcinoma. The importance of these factors is still the subject of intense research and debate.

Recent advances in the detection and treatment of prostate cancer lead to a far more optimistic outlook for the sexual health of those dealing with the disease. The evolution of new surgical techniques, new medical devices, medications, and traditional remedies will no doubt continue this healthier trend. One cover story in *Time Magazine* highlighted both the increasing rates of prostate cancer (both early and late stage) and the growing movement to seriously support the search for a cure. (As many as 80% of 80-year-old men were shown to have prostate cancer cells present at autopsy.)

Common Prostate Cancer Symptoms

- Urinary problems
- Inability to urinate, or difficulty starting or stopping the urine flow
- The need to urinate frequently, especially at night
- Weak or interrupted flow of urine
- Pain or burning during urination
- Difficulty having an erection
- Blood in the urine or semen
- Frequent pain in the lower back, hips, or upper thighs

In most cases, these symptoms are not due to prostate cancer. They may be caused by BPH, an infection, or another problem. However, a man with these symptoms should see a doctor so that any problem can be diagnosed and he can decide with his doctors guidance how he wants to treat the problem.

Sexually Transmitted Diseases: STD's

STD's still present a serious public health concern. Despite the fear of AIDS and the use of condoms, transmission rates are alarmingly high. The more partners you have, the more likely it is that you will contract a bacterial or viral sexually transmitted infection. Surveys reveal that 16% of men aged 18-59 paid for sex at some point in their lives, another potential source of infection.

Many STD's cause damage to the male reproductive tract if left untreated. Problems with fertility, for the man and his partner, can follow. That damage can also show up as a long-term infection that can make sex very uncomfortable. If you are sexually active and have been casual about using a condom, it's worth getting a regular blood test for STD's.

For Sex Problems, Prevention is the Best Cure

Prevention is the key to fighting any disease. While we can avoid certain behaviors or situations that may compromise our health, sometimes we face a health challenge that appears despite our best efforts to prevent it. The cause is often an inherited condition or tendency in your genes that no amount of vigilance, good diet, exercise, Eastern or Western medicine can eliminate.

Common among certain groups of men is the penchant to ignore or deny subtle changes that occur in their bodies. While there's no reason to become an alarmist, you should seek help and discuss health concerns with your partner, your family, and your physician. Doing so earlier rather than later can literally save your life! Often, the right therapies, diet, and supplements can turn many conditions around. But this requires your willingness to challenge yourself a little and, possibly, to make a few changes in your lifestyle so your body can do what it was designed to: maintain optimum health and balance throughout the seasons of life.

Creating an Environment that Promotes Good Sex

Somehow popular culture keeps alive the misguided myth that men should always "want it." However, the choices we make about our sex lives are dramatically affected by our social circumstances as well as other personal dynamics.

Opportunities for sex nowadays compete with many other factors—some of which relate to our being part of the world, and others which relate to our body's physiological readiness to engage. On top of all these, financial and time pressures may mean less opportunity for sex. Responsibilities for work, children, or a spouse can preoccupy us. Many men have difficulty navigating the stresses of dating and finding a compatible partner. For instance, you might not be attracted to many of the people you meet.

If you are in conflict with your partner, it's not unusual for sexual desire to diminish. Similarly, if social circumstances put you at odds with most of the people around you, your relations with sexual partners will be tainted.

Your sexual health doesn't exist in a vacuum. Enthusiasm and confidence can change dramatically with changes in work, living conditions, or the people around you. Fortunately, the opposite is also true: in an environment where you are valued, loved, and acknowledged, your self-respect and self-confidence will be greater, and you can draw upon them in your intimate encounters.

Recent biological studies even suggest that the presence of a long-term lover can increase the body's production of endorphins, the natural painkillers that give us a sense of serenity and security in our lives. One reason why it feels so horrible when we're abandoned or a lover dies is the reduction of these narcotic flashes that we're used to from the beloved just being around us.

> **TIPS**
>
> A common denominator in the life of many satisfied couples is playfulness. A sense of humor is an essential part of great sex taking the pressure off of any performance issues. Don't be afraid to laugh and have fun in the bedroom.

The cliché that sex in marriage is unsatisfying is contrary to what most people report. On the contrary, various studies show that married couples have better sex with one another than they have in affairs. Whether you're in a stable relationship or not, having a scintillating sex life means dealing with the unexpected, maintaining your own health and adjusting to your partner's moods and desires as the years pass.

Statistics show that men having healthy sexual relations in a secure relationship live longer and more enjoyably than single men. That enjoyment extends into their sex lives as well as other areas of work, relationship, and recreation.

Quite a few men find that they are attracted to, or interested in, relations with more than one woman, perhaps a shadow left from when we were more tribal creatures. Few men can fully love more than one woman at a time, however, and feel true serenity and security in their embrace. If you think you can, be prepared to spend a great deal of effort trying to accommodate and balance their energies and needs.

Relationships do not peak on the wedding night or on any other night. Rather, they wax and wane with the cycles of family, work, health and even nature. It is important to be aware of these cycles and to learn how to live harmoniously with them, in and out of the bedroom.

We know that cranes, among other species, choose their mates early and are bound to them for life. On the other side of the argument, however, there is what's become known as the "Coolidge Effect," from a story recounted about President Calvin Coolidge.

Mr. and Mrs. Coolidge were given separate tours while paying a visit to a farm. Mrs. Coolidge observed a rooster mounting a hen and asked how often this occurred. The answer was many times each day. "Please tell that to the President," said Mrs. Coolidge.

When the President was informed of the rooster's performance, he inquired if it was repeatedly with the same hen. "Oh, no," came the reply, "it's a different one each time."

"Tell that to Mrs. Coolidge," said the President!

Time And Love

We tend to think of aging as something that happens late in life, but the aging process begins at birth and sexuality changes every few years. Ultimately, changes that take place as you age may affect your sexual strength and stamina, paralleling changes in other physical abilities.

After 50, you probably find you need more direct stimulation of your genitals to get an erection than you did when you were younger. This is not because your sexual appetite or your attraction to your partner has disappeared, but because your body has naturally moved into a different "season." Erections will possibly become less firm and angle down more than when you were younger. The force of ejaculation is diminished and your recovery time is probably longer. Then again, you don't expect to run a marathon as fast or as far at 60 as you did at 20.

There are some positive differences between sex and sports with regard to aging: your ability in bed may actually improve. Older men can maintain an erection longer than before and thereby satisfy their partner more easily. You may discover more staying power and fewer "premature moments."

Also, don't assume that a woman's sexual appetite or ability diminishes as she ages: many women find that their interest in sex actually increases after

When many of us think of erections we tend to think the stiffer the better. But the truth is being hard enough for penetration is probably just fine. If you are concerned about blood flow or low testosterone issues the best time to check your erection is in the morning when the smooth muscles around the penis are relaxed allowing for easy engorgement. If you have trouble getting an erection in the morning you might be experiencing blood flow or testosterone issues.

menopause, perhaps because of their changing hormone levels. A cross-cultural survey has shown that sex is vitally important for older men in 70% of cultures and for older women in 80%.

In the East, Chinese masters of the art of love knew how to turn the seasons one more time, experiencing a second springtime in their old age. They knew that an active sex life is essential for counteracting the effects of aging, for maintaining one's health, and for living a longer, happier life.

Great news! Staying sexually active can actually help fight off impotence. Frequent erections mean frequent blood flow to the penis.

As we pass through our fifth, sixth, and seventh decades and beyond, coping with the changes we encounter in our bodies may take some mental and physical adjustment. Men in their 50s and older frequently comment that their erections are not as hard as they used to be. Physical and mental arousal is more difficult to achieve. Things that once easily produced erections—seeing your partner undressed, kissing or hugging, or even watching X-rated films—now no longer produce the same arousal. Men at this age often take longer to ejaculate, it may be a less forceful emission, and they don't have the need to ejaculate every time; every second or third time is more typical.

TIPS

As we age the time it takes us to reach a full erection and to reach orgasm may be a bit longer than in our younger days. But many men feel pressured to perform quickly in a sexual situation and are disappointed when their bodies don't react as the once did. Leading to, yes you guessed it, performance anxiety. But the good news is that the minimum sex session duration, not counting quickies, should be about 30 minutes. This is about the time needed for a woman to get fully aroused. So slow it down and take your time. You'll both be pleased with the results!

In other areas of our life we don't have the same outrageous expectations that we may inflict on our bodies. When it's old timers' day in baseball, we don't expect Rusty Staub and other stars of yesteryear to hit and run and catch like they used to. And we don't expect a 40-year-old man to run as fast as he did when he won the 100-meter race in the Olympics at age 22.

To the extent that we can rid ourselves of ridiculous expectations, accept our sexual parts in their current state, meet their needs, and enjoy sex for what it is and what it delivers to us … to that extent we can give and receive erotic pleasure as much as we want and for as long as we want.

To sum up...

- Testosterone level and potency decline naturally as men age.

- Maintaining physical fitness and good overall health can help a man perform better in the bedroom.

- Many external factors, especially stress and your relationship with your partner, affect libido and sex drive. Improving these factors (e.g., reducing stress, being more loving and open with your partner) can enhance sexual pleasure and performance.

The Truth about Erectile Dysfunction Drugs and Other Male Potency Cures

CHAPTER 2

"Sex is emotion in motion."

—Mae West

No doubt you've heard about, considered, or even tried the breakthrough erecticle dysfunction drugs since they hit the American marketplace. Perhaps you've had, or envied others for, positive experiences while using them. E.D. drugs have created a stir amongst the male (and female) population, not just for their assistance in bringing extinct volcanoes back to life, but also for the attention they have brought to the American view, denial, and celebration of their sexuality. Perhaps their most important side effect is the disclosure of many hidden fears, desires, and inadequacies about continued sexual pleasure for men in all age brackets.

Viagra, Levitra, and Cialis are all phosphodiesterase (PDE5) inhibitors—meaning they block ester linkages in phosphodiester compounds (see Appendix B). As we saw in Chapter 1, the physiology of erection involves the release of *nitric oxide* (*NO*) into the expanding corpus cavernosum during stimulation of the penis. This activates the enzyme guanylate cylase leading to an increase in levels of cyclic guanosine monophosphate (cGMP). The result is a smooth muscle relaxation in the corpus cavernosum and an increase of inflow of blood causing an erection. The E.D. drugs inhibit the type of PDE5 that is reposnible for breaking down the cGMP that builds up in the corpus cavernosum. Basically, the E.D. drugs enhance the effect of *NO* so that the blood does not leave but stays trapped there for longer than the body would normally allow.

The drugs help to open (dilate) the blood vessels, which is why caution is advised for anyone with cardiac, retina, headache, or circulatory problems. So the "back door" of the penis' circulation is closed, and those veins mentioned earlier—which allow blood to circulate out of the erect penis after a time—stay compressed. The result: the blood is forced to stay, freezing "Little Jimmy" in full salute. The erection is made easier and kept going longer.

> **CAUTION!**
>
> If you ever experience an erection that lasts more that 4 hours seek medical attention immediately. This condition, called priapism, is a possible side effect of some E.D. drugs. Priapism can lead to permanent damage to the penis, including the ability to have an erection.

FDA-approved package copy for the Viagra, Cialis, and Levitra all stress that at recommended doses the drugs have no effect in the absence of sexual stimulation. As one urologist explains, Viagra helps men who have a strong libido but have been unable to act on it. "There must be some activity that helps him get in the mood," insists this M.D. "If a male pops a pill but has not been properly stimulated, he will not be able to maintain function."

In the course of normal events when stimulation ceases, after ejaculation, or when the body isn't arousable for whatever organic reason, nitric oxide production fades and so does a man's erection. The body just isn't able to send energy into that area, often no matter how hard we try.

E.D. drugs, therefore, offer a targeted approach to men having problems getting erections or desiring an added boost to their banger. However, it does not at all address the underlying health issues of why the body is withholding sexual energy—stresses and imbalances that are diverting that essential energy into other organ systems that need it more.

When we hit our 40s and 50s, we just can't seem to get the engine running the way it did when it was newer or under less harsh conditions. If we think of the body as a somewhat closed system, like a car, we know that gas has to make it to the cylinders and not just get caught up in the carburetor in order to get us where we want to go. Likewise our body had priorities as to where the gas, our life energy, is needed most in order to keep us going.

How does it feel to take Viagra? I tried it months ago, because I wanted to know if I'd turn into a rampaging, ravaging 25-year-old stud. After taking half a dose (about 25 mg, I think), I waited. Sure enough, an hour later, my penis rose to a very erect position—but at the same time something felt not quite right: Though I had been stimulated by my mate, the "juiciness" and "aliveness" of my penile nerve endings that had usually accompanied stimulation and erection were missing.

It felt like a petrified log was attached to my loins. I wanted the real thing, and the drug wasn't giving it to me. I soon wanted this lack of feeling to go away...and I knew that it would take a while for the drug to wear off. I felt disappointed, and a little panicky.

My experience with Viagra is that it's almost an involuntary thing that happens to my physiology. You just give your penis the slightest bit of stimulation and it perks up. When I used it, there I was, with this big piece of lumber. All of the attendant parts—those aroused in cuddling and foreplay, and moved from Point A to Point Z in interaction with my mate—aren't required. With Viagra, they're simply not part of the process.

So for a pure hard-on, an E.D. drug might give the desired "lift." But it may not completely fulfill our wishes. If we want our bodies to regain optimal health and keep doing what comes naturally and continue to operate smoothly for the long term, then paying attention to the tuning, timing, and fuel to positively affect the whole vehicle may be necessary. There are no shortcuts to true sexual fulfillment.

Evolution of a Revolution

Viagra is a brand-name product manufactured by New York City-based Pfizer Pharmaceuticals.

Although Viagra is probably the most widely publicized pharmaceutical "sex pill," it was not the first. Several years before Viagra hit the market, Wellbutrin, an antidepressant manufactured by BurroughsWellcome, was found to have aphrodisiac qualities. In a test on 57 men and women with low sexual desire, 63% reported a rise in libido. But hope for usage in treating sexual dysfunction faded when Wellbutrin was found to trigger seizure activity in some patients.

Viagra was invented by a team of scientists, led by Dr. Ian Osterloh, at a Pfizer laboratory in England. As with Wellbutrin, Viagra was not originally invented for its current purpose as a sex pill.

Osterloh says his team was experimenting with treatments for angina and hypertension, not trying to invent a penis pill. To their surprise, the drug didn't lower blood pressure but did cause erections.

The name comes from a combination of the words "virility" (vi) and "Niagara" (agra). The cost of Viagra is about $10 a pill—approximately sixteen times the cost of the average herbal male potency supplement.

Clinical trials showed that 80% of 4,000 impotent men who took Viagra were able to achieve erections again. On March 27, 1998, the U.S. Food and Drug Administration (FDA) approved Viagra. During its first month on the market, April 1998, Viagra sales reached almost $100 million. Total sales of Viagra during its first nine months on the market totaled $788 million.

Overall, Pfizer's net income in 1998 increased 51% to $3.3 billion—$2.55 per share. Thanks in large part to Viagra's commercial success, sales for the entire pharmaceutical industry increased 35% worldwide in 1998. In response, pharmaceutical companies have expanded their sales forces by 40% to get doctors and pharmacies to recommend and carry their drugs.

An article in the New York *Daily News* proclaimed: "Viagra burst into the nation's bedrooms like a pharmaceutical supernova a year ago and set off a sexual revolution by rejuvenating legions of rundown Romeo's." *Playboy* magazine founder Hugh Hefner added, "It is as close as one can imagine to a Fountain of Youth."

So far, well over sixty million Viagra tablets have been sold. About one out of three U.S. doctors—225,000 M.D.s—have prescribed Viagra. More than four million Americans have taken Viagra; four out of ten are men age 50 or older.

To date, more than eight million prescriptions for Viagra have been written, mostly in the U.S. Viagra is approved by Medicaid in forty states; it is not covered by Medicare. A 1998 federal edict requires states to pay for Viagra "only when medically necessary."

Viagra is now sold in at least fifty countries worldwide. In Japan, Viagra approval took only a few months—remarkably fast compared with the thirty-five years it took for the Japanese government to approve use of the birth control pill as a contraceptive.

The Tide Turns

In May 1998, less than 2 months after Viagra went on the market, the *New York Times* (May 23, 1998) ran a story with the headline, "6 Taking Viagra Die, but the F.D.A. Draws No Conclusions." The article reported that six people taking the drug had died but that the Food and Drug Administration had no information linking, or not linking the deaths to the drug.

Just five days later, the *Daily News* ran a second Viagra story. This time the headline was "16 Took Viagra and Died – F.D.A.: No Link Yet, but Drug Eyed." According to the story, a total of sixteen men died after taking Viagra, including seven who died during or just after sex.

The FDA stressed that the clinical data on the deaths were incomplete. There was no evidence that Viagra was the cause. The deaths did not, according to an FDA report, change the FDA's perspectives on the safety of this approved pharmaceutical.

Then, in November 1998, the FDA required Pfizer to add new statements to its warning label. The label already warned that Viagra should not be taken with nitrate-containing medicine, such as nitroglycerine; the combination can cause a potentially fatal drop in blood pressure.

Now the warning label also states that the FDA has received reports of heart attacks, sudden cardiac death, and hypertension among Viagra users. It also advises doctors to be cautious about prescribing Viagra for men who have had a heart attack, stroke, life-threatening arrhythmia, significantly low or high blood pressure, history of cardiac failure, or the eye disease retinitis pigmentosa.

As this book went to press, close to 130 deaths, mostly men with heart conditions, are being investigated for links to Viagra. The American Heart Association warns against Viagra usage for men who take medicine for high blood pressure.

"Don't take Viagra if you're also taking nitrates for heart disease," advises Dr. Stephen Sinatra, a cardiologist. Together, the two substances can result in a dangerous drop in blood pressure. "You may even become dizzy and pass out," Sinatra warns.

There have been other problems with Viagra. Clinical studies show it does not work in 30% of men, especially those with circulatory system problems. Sometimes the erections last too long—hours at a time—becoming a nuisance and painful.

The Federal Aviation Administration (FAA) recommends that pilots not take Viagra for six hours or longer before flights. The drug, which can affect vision, can affect pilots' ability to distinguish the colors of control panel and runway lights.

Some sex professionals even see Viagra's effectiveness (remember, for seven out of ten men, it works!) as a liability in itself. They feel that Viagra's emphasis on erection, penetration, and orgasm is perhaps to the detriment of the relationship side of sex. A T-shirt sold in the Harriet Carter mail order catalog jokingly refers to Viagra as "an exciting new drug that increases blood flow to a man's brain"—a sarcastic reference to the belief that many men do their thinking with their dorkal hoses.

"Sex isn't just about making physical connections," says sex therapist Greg McGreer. "If the ability to make an emotional relationship is poor, the ability to perform sexually also will be poor." Robert Butler, president of the International Longevity Center at Mt. Sinai Medical Center, adds, "Viagra is neither an aphrodisiac nor a love potion for a relationship that's in distress."

"Don't believe the lies that say sexual intimacy becomes extinct in old age," says Dr. Douglas E. Rosenau. "By physical necessity, it may change. But emotionally and spiritually, it just gets better."

The Soft Side of Sex with E.D. Drugs

E.D. drugs can enable men who are impotent to once again achieve an erection, fairly easily. But, as scientists and consumers point out, it does not boost libido or desire. Most herbal potency supplements contain multiple ingredients. Some address erectile dysfunction, while others intensify sex drive, desire, and energy. Therefore, herbal supplements can provide a holistic path to better sex, while E.D. drugs only address it from the waist down.

"Viagra does not affect a male's libido," states the manager of a urology group in the Northwest that treats men with erectile dysfunction. "A male with no interest in sexual activity will not develop an interest if he takes this drug."

Other Potency Technologies

In addition to drugs, the medical establishment offers a number of other technologies for treating erectile dysfunction:

- Penile injections involve injecting an erection-inducing drug directly into the base of your penis. The most commonly used agents include papverine, phentolamine, and prostaglandin E. Injections should not be done more than twice a week.

- One injectable product, Caverject, was the first prescription medicine to receive FDA approval for treating erectile dysfunction. Made by Upjohn, Caverject is a dose of prostaglandin injected into the penis using a needle. It works by preventing the breakdown of a brain chemical that helps open penile arteries, so blood vessels can dilate. This increases blood flow to the penis, allowing erectile tissue to stiffen.

- Muse (Medicated Urethral System for Erection) is a tiny suppository inserted into the urethra. It contains the same medication as Caverjet. Launched in 1996 by Vivus Inc., Muse sales were $130 million in 1997, but declined dramatically in 1998 when Viagra was introduced to the public. Muse has a good safety record, with just one recorded patient death in over a million prescriptions.

- A variety of tubes and rings have been designed to solve the problem of erectile dysfunction. Penis rings are rubber-band-like devices placed at the base of the penis. They constrict the penis, keeping blood in the shaft to prevent erection-forming blood from leaving the organ. The Rejoyn Support Sleeve is a soft rubber tube available in pharmacies without a prescription. Placed over the penis, the tube is supposed to give sufficient rigidity to permit intercourse.

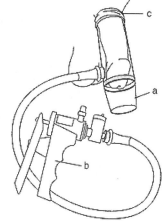

Figure 3: The Penis Pump

A vaccum-constricting device causes an erection by creating a partial vacuum around the penis, drawing blood into the corpus cavernosum. In this illustration you will see (a) the plastic cylinder, which slides over the penis, (b) a pump that is used to draw air out of the cylinder, and (c) an elastic ring which fits over the base of the penis trapping the blood and sustaining the erection when the cylinder is removed. (Image courtesy of NIH)

- Penis pumps (see Figure 3), similar in design to hand-operated breast pumps for women, are plastic cylinders that can be placed over the penis. Pumping by hand forms a vacuum, withdrawing air around the penis. Under pressure, blood flows rapidly into the penis to form an erection. Once the erection takes place, a penis ring can be put around the base to maintain the hard-on. The ring should not be left on for more than a half hour.

■ A medical doctor can prescribe and treat you with testosterone injections. These are administered via intra-muscular injection or through skin patches. According to the *USP DI*, a drug directory published by Medical Economics, the danger is that male hormone injections in a patient with normal testosterone can stimulate prostate growth, cause liver damage or tumors, stop sperm production, cause skin problems, and even promote prostate cancer.

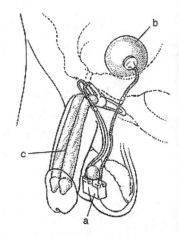

Figure 4: The Inflatable Penile Implant

With an inflatable implant, erection is achieved by squeezing a small pump that is implanted in a scrotum. The pump causes fluid to flow from a reservoir (b) residing in the lower pelvis to two cylinders (c) residing in the penis. The cylinders expand to create the erection. (Image courtesy of NIH)

■ Depending on the root cause of the problem (pun intended), a surgeon can use a penile implant. These are prosthetic devices surgically inserted into the corpus cavernosa (spongy chambers) of the penis. To date, more than 250,000 men in the U.S. have had penile implants. Semi-rigid implants stay hard all the time, but are not fully erect, so embarrassment and inconvenience are avoided. Another option is to implant an inflatable cylinder into the penis (see Figure 4). You or your partner can hand-pump the cylinder when an erection is desired. The pump and reservoir are usually implanted unobtrusively in the scrotum or abdomen. To get an erection, squeeze the pump. Fluid in the reservoir

Despite the unpleasant imagery penile surgery and implantation conjures, many men will go to almost any length (pun again intended) to regain the ability to have an erection. One article in the New York *Daily News* reported that a New York woman convinced her lover to pose as her husband so family insurance would cover the boyfriend's $15,000 penile implant. Incidentally, the article reports that the boyfriend had tried Viagra "but experienced an erection that wouldn't go away and wound up in the emergency room."

flows into the cylinder implanted in the penile shaft, causing it to extend and harden. Another squeeze activates a release ring that lets fluid drain back into the reservoir, deflating the erection.

- Varicoceles (blocked veins in the groin region similar to varicose veins in the legs) and other vascular conditions sometimes cause impotence in younger men; these can also be corrected by penile microsurgery (revascularization).

To sum up...

- Although over 130 deaths, mostly men with heart conditions, may be linked to taking the drug, Viagra has <u>not</u> been proven as the direct cause of their deaths.

- Erectile dysfunction drugs cause a stiff erection but do not enhance desire, libido, or pleasure, nor do they have aphrodisiac properties.

- E.D. drugs are not the only conventional medical alternatives for treating erectile dysfunction; others include penile injections, devices, penile implants, microsurgery, and testosterone therapy.

3 Natural Alternatives to E.D. Drugs—an A – Z Guide

*"Is it not strange that desire
should so many years outlive
performance?"*

—William Shakespeare

Although Americans now spend $30 billion annually on nutritional supplements, the idea of consuming natural substances for healing goes back to Biblical times: *Psalm CIV* says of the Lord, "He causeth the herb to grow for the service of man." And 2,500 years ago, Hippocrates counseled, "Let food be thy medicine, and medicine thy food."

Using nature's incredible healing power is nothing new. Did you know that thousands of years ago, the ancient Chinese and Egyptians used herbs like ginger and garlic to keep themselves healthy?

Examples of herbal healing abound. For instance, the 5,000-year-old Ayurdevic texts of ancient India recommend guggul, a gummy resin from the Boswellia tree, for a variety of conditions including arthritis, diarrhea, and pulmonary disease.

Or consider the growing popularity of St. John's Wort. From the ancient Greeks through the Middle Ages, St. John's Wort has been used as a practical folk remedy for treating kidney problems, healing wounds, and alleviating nervous disorders. Annual sales of St. John's Wort now exceed $200 million.

In the 1500s, cinchona (Indian fever bark) was used to treat malaria and other fever-inducing diseases. More recently, another plant, bilberry, was given to Royal Air Force pilots to improve their night vision when flying night-time missions during World War II.

Even the pharmaceutical industry recognizes the healing power of plants, although they don't widely acknowledge it. Did you know, for example, that 25 percent of Western pharmaceuticals contain ingredients from plants found in the rain forest?

Most people don't realize so many drugs are derived from plants, because pharmaceutical companies don't advertise this fact—after all, they make a lot of money selling their prescription medicines. But a few years ago, researchers at Roche Vitamin Laboratories published a study on the benefits of supplementation. Their findings: if all women of childbearing age were to supplement with zinc and folic acid, and all people over 50 took vitamin E, the annual savings in the U.S. in hospital charges alone would be nearly $20 billion.

"Many people, both men and women, are now taking herbal products," Ann Landers wrote in her syndicated column, in response to a reader who wanted to know if it is safe to take Viagra. "They are less expensive than prescription drugs and have fewer side effects, and the results have apparently been very satisfactory." According to an article in *Prevention*, Americans now make at least 629 million visits to alternative practitioners annually vs. 386 million visits annually to family doctors. According to a study published in the *Journal of the American Medical Association*, four out of ten Americans have tried alternative medicine.

There is a great deal of information available about herbs, vitamins, minerals and foods that are believed to strengthen the male reproductive tract and lead to a more satisfying sex life. In this area, science and research are constantly evolving. New vitamins, minerals, amino acids and herbs will no doubt appear which will complement those mentioned here. This chapter provides a layman's overview of the most widely used and proven natural nutrients known to enhance male sexual potency, overall health, vitality, and performance.

Alfalfa (Medicago sativae)

If you are old enough (like I am), the name alfalfa may bring back memories of the TV show *The Little Rascals* and the singing boy with the slicked-back hair. Or, you might instead think of a stringy sprout you find in your sandwiches and salads in restaurants. But in fact, alfalfa may prove to help you in quite unexpected, and quite desirable, ways.

As we've discussed, erections require blood flow to the penis. So the more the body's blood flow is compromised, the more likely you are to have problems getting an erection.

Atherosclerosis, a common type of arteriosclerosis (thickening of the arterial walls), is a major cause of impotence. In atherosclerosis, atheromas – a yellow plaque containing cholesterol, lipoids, and lipophages – collect inside the arteries, blocking blood flow.

That's what makes alfalfa such an attractive nutrient for men worried about getting it up for sex. Animal studies have shown that alfalfa helps prevent these plaque deposits and lower cholesterol, protecting you against atherosclerosis, stroke, and heart disease.

Also known as lucerne, alfalfa is a fodder plant native to southwestern Asia. The root system goes as deep as 30 feet, enabling the alfalfa plants to survive periods of extreme drought.

The ancient Chinese used alfalfa to stimulate appetite and treat ulcers and other digestive ailment. Ayurvedic physicians in ancient India prescribed alfalfa for arthritis pain and fluid retention.

Later, early American pioneers used alfalfa to treat boils, scurvy, urinary and bowel problems, and cancer (a study published in the Journal of the National Cancer Institute shows that alfalfa binds carcinogens in the colon and helps speed their elimination from the body). Herbalists promote alfalfa as a detoxifier for cleaning the liver and blood stream.

Alfalfa contains no fat, no sodium, and few calories. But it *does* contain chlorophyll, beta carotene, vitamin A, vitamin B_6, vitamin D, vitamin E, calcium, phosphorous, vitamin K, saponins, and essential amino acids.

The obvious source of alfalfa is to eat those stringy sprouts some of us move to the side of our plate. The sprouts, which should be eaten raw, go great with most meals, either on sandwiches or as a side dish drizzled with a little soy sauce.

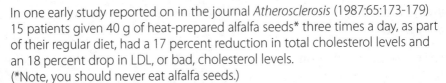
STUDY RESULTS

In one early study reported on in the journal *Atherosclerosis* (1987:65:173-179) 15 patients given 40 g of heat-prepared alfalfa seeds* three times a day, as part of their regular diet, had a 17 percent reduction in total cholesterol levels and an 18 percent drop in LDL, or bad, cholesterol levels.
(*Note, you should never eat alfalfa seeds.)

(Molgaard J., et al "Alfalfa seeds lower low density lipoprotein cholesterol..." Atherosclerosis 1987;65:173-179)

Atherosclerosis. 1987 May;65(1-2):173-9.

Alfalfa seeds lower low density lipoprotein cholesterol and apolipoprotein B concentrations in patients with type II hyperlipoproteinemia.

Molgaard J, von Schenck H, Olsson AG.

Fifteen patients with hyper-lipoproteinemia (HLP), types IIA (n = 8), IIB (n = 3) and IV (n = 4) were given 40 g of heat prepared alfalfa seeds 3 times daily at mealtimes for 8 weeks with otherwise unchanged diet. In patients with type II HLP alfalfa treatment caused after 8 weeks a maximal lowering of pretreatment median values of total plasma cholesterol from 9.58 to 8.00 mmol/l (P less than 0.001) and low density lipoprotein (LDL) cholesterol from 7.69 to 6.33 mmol/l (P less than 0.01), which corresponds to decreases of 17% and 18%, respectively. Maximal decrease was 26% in total cholesterol and 30% in LDL cholesterol. In two patients with hypercholesterolemia the LDL cholesterol decreased less than 5%. Apolipoprotein B decreased in the same period from 2.17 to 1.43 g/l (P less than 0.05) in type II HLP, corresponding to 34% decrease, whereas apolipoprotein A-I did not change. Body weight increased slightly during the first 4 weeks of alfalfa treatment (P less than 0.001) probably because of the caloric content in the alfalfa seeds. After cessation of treatment, all lipoprotein concentrations returned to pretreatment levels. We conclude that alfalfa seeds can be added to the diet to help normalize serum cholesterol concentrations in patients with type II HLP.

PMID: 3606731
[PubMed - indexed for MEDLINE]

A number of incidents of food poisoning related to salmonella and e.coli have been linked to commercially grown alfalfa sprouts in several years. The Centers for Disease Control and Prevention (CDC) advise that the elderly, young children, and anyone with a compromised immune system not eat these sprouts. According to an article in *Consumer Reports* (October 1999, p. 61), more than 1,000 Americans fell ill between 1995 and 1999 in nearly a dozen outbreaks involving contaminated sprouts.

Growing your own alfalfa at home, under controlled conditions, can bypass this health hazard. Alfalfa *seeds* should not be eaten under any circumstances.

The safest route is to take nutritional supplements made out of alfalfa leaves, which are higher in the important nutrients that make alfalfa so desirable. The leaves contain l-canaverine, a non-protein amino acid shown in animal studies to be effective against leukemia and cancer cells.

Dosage: 50 milligrams (mg) daily. Infusion: Add 1 to 2 teaspoons of dried leaves per cup of boiling water, steep for 10 to 20 minutes, drink 3 cups daily.

Grow your own alfalfa!

Buy and rinse alfalfa seeds under cold water in a colander. Place in a jar. Secure cheese-cloth to the jar with a rubber band. Rinse seeds again, letting water drain through the cloth. Refill the jar with water and soak seeds overnight.

The next morning, tilt the jar on its side and let the water drain. Gently shake the jar to spread the seeds along the side.

Lay the jar on a towel in a cool, dark cupboard. Fill and drain the jar thoroughly two or three times daily. When tiny leaves begin to show on the ends of the sprouts, place them in indirect light for a few hours. The leaves will turn green with chlorophyll. Store the sprouts in a closed container in the refrigerator. Use within five days.

—Janit London, "Sprouts for Your Sprout,"
Inner Realm magazine.

Asparagus root

I couldn't find much detailed information about this herb, and eating this yummy vegetable while praying for inspiration didn't seem to help. Because of the phallic shape of the shoots it has long been regarding as an aphrodisiac. In fact the Ayurvedic name for it, Shatavari, is reported to mean literally "she who has one hundred husbands." In Traditional Chinese Medicine it is said to increase feelings of love and compassion. In India the herb is administered to promote fertility, among other things. The steroidal glycosides in the herb can effect hormone production and may be responsible for its rumored good-emotion-influencing abilities.

We do know that asparagus root is an anti-inflammatory and a diuretic. It has

STUDY RESULTS

According to an early study published in the *British Medical Journal* the pungent odor of urine after eating asparagus that was once thought to be an inborn error of metabolism has been proven to actually be a specific smell hypersensitivity. It turns out if you can smell the odor in your own urine you can smell it in anyone's urine who has eaten asparagus.

Br Med J. 1980 Dec 20-27;281(6256):1676-8.

A polymorphism of the ability to smell urinary metabolites of asparagus.

Lison M, Blondheim SH, Melmed RN.

The urinary excretion of (an) odorous substance(s) after eating asparagus is not an inborn error of metabolism as has been supposed. The detection of the odour constitutes a specific smell hypersensitivity. Those who could smell the odour in their own urine could all smell it in the urine of anyone who had eaten asparagus, whether or not that person was able to smell it himself. Thresholds for detecting the odour appeared to be bimodal in distribution, with 10% of 307 subjects tested able to smell it at high dilutions, suggesting a genetically determined specific hypersensitivity.

PMID: 7448566
[PubMed - indexed for MEDLINE]

been used to treat diseases of the urinary tract. It has also been shown to effectively treat kidney conditions including, most commonly kidney stones.

In a 1991 study conducted at the Shandong Provincial Hospital of Traditional Chinese Medicine, 413 impotent males were given an herbal formulation consisting of asparagus root, epimedium, and astralagus. Within 72 days, almost six out of ten patients were completely cured and could attain a normal erection.

In another study, this one conducted at the Xiamen International Center for Traditional Chinese Medicine Research, 120 men suffering from sexual dysfunction were given a supplement containing asparagus root, wild yam, and cuscatae. Approximately 42 percent said they were completely cured.

Asparagus root is best consumed as a tea, by cutting the root for preparation. The optimum daily dosage is 45-60 grams (g) of rhizome (root), or equivalent preparations.

Astragalus

The two best things about astragalus is that it may help you become a father (assuming you're trying) and it will likely strengthen the immune system. A 1992 National Yang-Ming Medical College (Taiwan) study suggests that astragalus stimulates sperm motility, which means it will make your little guys move more easily. Since low motility is a common cause of infertility in men, this root may prove to create a lot of proud papas.

If you have a cold, cancer, or any number of other ailments for which your own precious immune system is failing you, astragalus may help you too. Used since ancient times in traditional Chinese medicine, this sweet, warm substance is considered to be an ideal treatment, and in most minor cases a perfect remedy for anyone who has difficulty with his immune system in any way. Sometimes called locoweed, it is more commonly known in English as milk root.

Astragalus also has many other uses, including treatment of heart congestive failure and depleted red blood cell formation in the bone marrow.

DID YOU KNOW?

In your lifetime your testicles will produce an average of fourteen gallons ejaculate.

The majority of ejaculate is made up of fructose, the same sugar found in a glass of juice.

Particularly in Chinese culture, it has been used to treat fatigue, excessive sweating, frequent colds and shortness of breath, as well as various ailments of the urinary canal and anus. It has been found to promote general healing throughout the bodily systems. In one Chinese study, patients injected with astragalus extract for 3 to 4 months showed increased production of their body's antiviral compounds alpha and gamma-interferon.

Astragalus can be used with ginseng to counteract debility, decreased appetite, fatigue, or excessive sweating. In addition astragalus has been shown to widen blood vessels and increase blood flow, which has some obvious benefits for both our hearts and our sexual organs.

In a study conducted at Zhejiang Provincial Hospital of Chinese Medicine, 182 men suffering from low sperm count were given an herbal formula including astragalus, cuscutae, and epimedium. More than a third were reported to be completely cured.

Preparations and dosage: put 1 teaspoon of the root into 1 cup of water, bring to a boil and simmer for 10-15 minutes. Drink 3 times daily. Tincture: take 2-4 milliliters (ml) of the tincture 3 times a day.

Avena Sativa/Wild Oats

How often do you hear that eating a common breakfast food can reduce stress, calm your nerves, increase performance, endurance, and metabolism, counteract effects of old age, and help your sex life? (Okay, but how often are those claims actually true?)

You probably didn't realize that "sowing your wild oats" was a phrase based in fact; wild oats have been used for their aphrodisiac (as well as other healing) properties in Europe for centuries. Stallions fed wild oats supposedly become more libidinous.

In 1985, The Institute for Advanced Study of Human Sexuality gave 9 men and 10 women ages 22 to 64 daily doses of 300 mg avena sativa for 4 weeks. Women reported a 21 percent increase in sexual thoughts and fantasies, a 19 percent increase in sexual satisfaction, and a 30 percent increase in frequency of sexual intercourse. Men reported a 25 percent increase in sexual

Oats have long been used by breeders to help boost the libido and fertility of their male animals. Giving new meaning to the term "sow your wild oats".

gratification and a 22 percent increase in genital sensitivity.

Avena sativa refers to the entire oat plant. *Avena fructus* refers to the fruit. *Avena herba* is the leafy part of the plant. Wild oats are considered a "nervine," meaning that the grain calms the nervous system. It is thus an unusual substance, proving to be both stimulating and relaxing at once. I'm not sure how that works, but both effects are firmly grounded in western empirical study.

(Avena sativa is not the only plant known to have both calming and stimulating effects. Different varieties of ginseng similarly have the ability to either calm or stimulate.)

Wild oats are regularly used for ailments of the intestinal tract, acute and chronic anxiety, stress, and weakness of the bladder. It has been used for diseases and discomforts due to old age, for the healing and treatment of pulled or strained muscles, as a remedy against tobacco abuse, and to increase endurance and performance capacity.

Wild oats have been used traditionally for external skin treatments of various kinds, and internally for skin and bones. They are said to be a sleeping aid.

> **TIPS**
>
> Wild oat extracts have been used in India to help ease opium addictions. One study showed that wild oats were effective in reducing cigarette withdrawal symptoms. So if you are giving up smoking you might want to try a wild oats extract to ease the cravings.

In combination with other herbs, wild oats have been used to treat heart ailments, for general circulatory difficulties, and to treat weakness and fatigue.

Dosage: For treatment of ailments (as opposed to breakfast), 3 grams can be brewed with/liter boiling water for tea. If you can find the fluid extract, 10-30 drops can be used daily. You might experiment with this one: since toxicity isn't a problem, you can safely test the herb's effects on your system in various amounts. But to be safe, as always, consult your doctor first.

Bee Pollen and Flower Pollen

I like to think that there's something suggestive about the fact that bee pollen is made from the juices of male flowers—for instance, an inter-natural exchange of potency. But the truth is that this substance, made of flower pollen and mixed with the bee's own honey, packs enough nutritive substance that it works by boosting our overall inner-workings, thereby supporting the individual processes that we consider most important (like sexual activity!).

Bee pollen is known as a complete food, balanced with vitamins, minerals, proteins, carbohydrates, fats, enzyme precursors, and all essential amino acids. It is great for anyone with extra nutritional or energy needs, and due to its superfood quality, it supports most of our bodily systems. Among these is the endocrine system, aiding in our production of hormones. It therefore is thought to treat various prostate-related problems and ailments. In fact, used in conjunction with pumpkin seeds and nettle root, bee pollen has been shown to reduce enlarged prostate glands in men suffering from benign prostate hyperplasia (BPH).

Bee pollen, or propolis, is a multifunctional material used by bees in the construction and maintenance of their hives. Recent studies also suggest that pollen reduces the signs of aging, augmenting both mental and physical activity. It has been proven good for the skin, and is used to fight bacteria, fungus, virus, and tumor development in the body. It also boosts the body's natural antioxidant, blood production, and cardiovascular systems.

CAUTION!

Some people can have an allergic reaction to bee products so be sure to start with a small amount. Be on the lookout for allergic symptoms like an itchy throat, flushed skin, headaches or wheezing. As always it's best to consult with a doctor before taking any new supplement.

Closely related to bee pollen is flower pollen (of course, it is the same thing without the interaction with the bee). Flower pollen, too, has shown to aid people suffering from BPH.

A study published in the *Journal of Urology* concluded that flower pollen extract (the name brand used was Cernilton) taken over a six month period resulted in improvement in 70 percent of cases. These patients showed a significant decrease in residual urine and, in fact, a marked decrease in the diameter of the prostate gland.

Cernilton has been used extensively in Europe to treat prostatitis. In addition it has been found to have a relaxing effect on the urethra.

Dosage: The usual dose is two teaspoons daily. Look for "unsprayed" pollen in the health food stores (meaning the plants haven't been treated with pesticides or other chemicals).

Burdock

Burdock might be a good choice if you have anything that's inflamed or irritated. It has been shown to aid in kidney function, but it has many other uses as well.

Burdock is often used as an anti-inflammatory, and reportedly removes impurities and waste products of many sorts that may be stuck in your kidneys, skin, or mucous and serous membranes. By doing so, burdock can help move your body to a state of integration and good health.

Aside from these benefits, burdock has been used to treat skin ailments of various sorts, digestive problems, and most bodily functions that involve ridding the body of any unwanted substance (like coughing does). Skin conditions burdock can treat include dry or scaly skin, dandruff, and psoriasis if used over long periods of time. For treating skin problems, burdock may be combined with yellow dock, red clover, or cleavers.

Burdock may be used as a compress for wounds and ulcers, and externally or internally for eruptions on the head, face, and neck. It is also effective as a diuretic, and reports suggest the effective treatment of rheumatism, gout and sciatica, and the relief of syphilitic conditions.

Preparation and dosage: put 1 teaspoon in 1 cup of water, bring to boil, let simmer for 10-15 minutes. Drink 3 times daily. Tincture: take 2-4 ml 3 times a day. Burdock may also be used as a compress or poultice for external application to irritated areas of the skin.

Calcium Citrate

If after eating a chicken drum stick, you try to bend the bone, you'll find you can't. It's stiff, and that's because of the calcium it contains.

To prove this, put the bone in a jar containing a mixture of half water and half vinegar; let it soak for a few days. Now remove the bone and try to bend it. Amazingly, you'll find the bone, leached of its calcium, is amazingly flexible and pliable; if it's long enough, you'll even be able to tie a knot in it!

Your body contains a lot of calcium – about 2 fi pounds–and 99 percent of it can be found in your bones and teeth. The other 1 percent is in the bloodstream and fluid surrounding your cells.

And here's the problem: Your bones act as a sort of "calcium warehouse" for your body. When you don't get enough calcium, the body determines that it's more important for the bloodstream and cells to maintain their calcium levels than the bones. So calcium is removed from the skeleton and transferred to the cells. If this calcium deficiency continues over a long period of time, your bones lose too much calcium, making them fragile and prone to fracture.

CAUTION!

If you have thyroid or kidney disease be sure to check with your doctor before taking calcium.

TIPS

Since calcium cannot be absorbed without vitamin D be sure to get some natural sunlight to stock up on this sunshine vitamin. Also keep in mind that our body's ability to convert sunlight into vitamin D tends to decline as we age. So you might want to consider a vitamin D supplement. If you prefer there are calcium supplements that already contain vitamin D that will make adding both nutrients to your diet easy.

You can now readily see why calcium is an important supplement for us as we age to avoid bone loss that can lead to brittleness and osteoporosis. A study presented at the Second Joint Meeting of the American Society for Bone and Mineral Research and the International Bone and Mineral Society reported on a group of subjects who took 400 mg of elemental calcium twice a day. After 2 years, their bone density was significantly higher than a control group not taking the calcium supplements.

In addition to serving as a basic building block of strong bones, calcium maintains muscular growth and helps regulate heartbeat. It maintains the integrity of cell membranes and capillaries, and also enhances transmission of nerve impulses, renal function, respiration, and blood coagulation. In a study published in the *New England Journal of Medicine* taking 1200 mg daily of calcium reduced colorectal adenomas, which are precursors of colon cancer, by 24 percent.

You've no doubt seen the TV commercials that proclaim, "Milk—it does a body good." One of the best things about milk is its high calcium content. However, a growing group of experts now question whether or not the calcium in milk is as easily absorbed by the body after it goes through the pasteurization process. The jury is still out on this one. Luckily, their are other foods that are rich in calcium as well including yogurt, cheese, salmon, sardines, clams, oysters, shrimp, kale, broccoli, soybeans, tofu, collard greens, turnip greens, and mustard greens.

As far as supplements, I think calcium citrate is the way to go. It is more easily absorbed than other forms of calcium. And since it can be digested without stomach acids, there are fewer gastrointestinal side effects.

Suggested dosage: 250 to 750 mg of calcium citrate daily.

Cayenne

Those of you who use chili pepper, red pepper, paprika, or hot pepper sauce already have a relationship with this herb. You know that it's spice makes your mouth feel alive—but due to its power as a stimulant and ability to increase blood flow, if taken in the right doses it can make your loins feel alive too. The main ingredient in cayenne causing these sensations is known pharmacologically as capsicum.

Many people believe pepper to be a sexual stimulant. In 1970, following an outbreak of sexual offenses in prisons, the Peruvian government banned the serving of hot pepper sauces in prison cafeterias, claiming that they aroused sexual desires and were therefore inappropriate fare. The Turks have long used crushed red peppers in love potions.

Brahmacharya, the principles for attainment of purity of soul and body, forbid India's young Brahmans from eating hot peppers. The peppers were believed to produce too much heat in the body system, making blood and sexual fluids watery and the mind restless.

David Livingstone, of Stanley and Livingston fame, reported that native African women bathed in water spiced with dissolved pepper juice to make themselves more attractive to the opposite sex. In medieval India, pepper was used as an aid in bringing women to orgasm.

Cayenne is primarily used in medicine as a powerful stimulant to increase blood flow and circulation to all parts of the body. In addition to stimulating your sex organs, it strengthens the heart, arteries, capillaries and nerves. Hot peppers are also used to treat depression, debility, lack of energy, and any condition caused by reduced blood flow. In addition, cayenne is thought by some to lower cholesterol, triglycerides, and blood pressure, and has been found in certain patients to be an anti-carcinogen.

Topical creams and ointments made with capsicum are used to treat nerve pain from shingles, diabetes, and surgery and have been shown very effective for arthritic pain. Clinical studies have shown that as many as 80 percent of arthritis sufferers experienced significant pain relief with topical capsaicin. Pain relief occurs almost immediately after the cream is applied to the afflicted area. Published research indicates that capsaicin reduces joint inflammation and the sensitivity of nerves.

Cayenne's medicinal uses are documented in the United States, Europe, China, and India. It has been used to stimulate the digestive system, to reduce flatulence, both internally and externally to treat cold hands and feet and sore muscles or joints, and in select Native American cultures as a stimulant and to wean children.

Dosage: Usual dosage is 5-15 drops, or 60 mg, of tincture. You may also mix a teaspoon with a cup of boiling water, let it infuse for ten minutes or so, and drink a tablespoon of the infusion with water as often as you like.

Warning: Cayenne is an irritant. Large doses can me harmful to mucus membranes and to the gastro-intestinal tract. Toxicity has resulted in animals in doses of 0.5 µg/kg body weight. It may interfere with antihypertensive therapy.

Chromium

You've no doubt seen advertisements for chromium picolinate, a nutritional supplement promoted for weight loss. Chromium increases your metabolism. Some experts believe that when taking chromium you may be able to burn calories faster instead of storing those calories as unhealthy body fat. As a bonus for dieters, many users report chromium reduces the appetite and craving for sweets.

In a double-blind randomized study, slightly overweight patients were given 200 to 400 mcg chromium picolinate daily. After 72 days, these patients had lost body fat and gained muscle mass compared to a control group taking only a placebo. Subsequent studies have not repeated these exact results and the debate continues.

But even if you're not trying to shed a few pounds, chromium is essential for a healthy body. It has been shown to lower cholesterol and control blood sugar levels in diabetics.

Your body does not manufacture chromium, so you need to take it in through foods or supplements, or both. As we age chromium deficiencies are thought to be more common. Unfortunately, there is no test the doctor can give you to determine whether you have a chromium deficiency.

The human body has difficulty absorbing chromium, so it may be best taken in a compound such as chromium asparate or chromium picolinate. Once chromium is converted into its biologically active form in your body, it helps insulin metabolize fat, use protein, and convert sugar into energy. In 14 out of 17 clinical studies, chromium has been shown to control glucose levels in diabetic patients and others with high blood glucose levels. Recall from chapter 1 that diabetic men, more than any other group, suffer from impotence. Control the diabetes, and you improve your chances of overcoming impotence.

In a recent collaborative study between the U.S. Human Nutrition Research Center and Beijing Medical University, adults with diabetes were given from 100 to 500 mcg daily chromium picolinate. Their blood glucose, insulin levels, cholesterol, and glycated hemoglobin (a measure of blood sugar control) decreased moderately vs. a control group given only a placebo.

> **CAUTION !**
>
> If you are diabetic be sure to consult your doctor before you start taking chromium. The mineral may cause your blood sugar levels to even out making it necessary to adjust your medications.

Foods containing chromium include mushrooms, oysters, clams, wheat germ, cheese, lentils, turkey, chicken, wine, apples, strawberries, brewer's yeast, pork, brown rice, wheat bread, meat, liver, cereal, corn oil, cottage cheese, broccoli, and spinach. Since the soil in the United States often has an inadequate supply of chromium, our crops are often lower in chromium than they should be. Modern food processing techniques can also rob grains, cereals, sugar cane, and other foods of their chromium content.

> **S**everal studies seem to indicate that zinc negatively affects chromium absorption. If you are taking zinc and chromium at the same time you may not be getting the full benefits from your chromium supplement.

Official U.S. RDA is 50 to 200 mcg daily for adults.

Cobalamin (Vitamin B$_{12}$)

This vitamin will sound to you a lot like Vitamin B$_6$ (see below) but this does one key male-important thing that B$_6$ does not do—it can raise your sperm count.

One of the numerous bodily functions in which B$_{12}$ takes part is fertility; it is a nutrient necessary for the fertility of both men and women. A deficiency of B_{12} leads to a reduction in the number and potency of sperm, while a supplement even in healthy men can lead to an increase in sperm count and motility (that's the ability for the little buggers to move toward their goal).

But while you get some help with becoming a father (assuming you are seeking that sort of help) why not also gain energy, reduce fatigue or depression, and increase concentration? Cobalamin, the clinical term for B_{12}, is necessary for DNA replication, red blood cell production, and the transmission of nervous impulses. Numerous emotional and mental processes rely on sufficient levels of it, and it has been shown to effectively treat depression and loss of cognitive ability due to age.

TIPS

If you want to maximize your vitamin B_{12} intake, don't microwave your food. A study printed in the *Journal of Agricultural and Food Chemistry* showed that beef and pork lose 30 to 40 percent of their active vitamin B_{12} when microwaved.

Vitamin B_{12} protects the myelin coating that surrounds your nerves, preventing nerve deterioration that can cause loss of memory and other vital brain functions. The American Medical Association reports that vitamin B_{12} is important in the production of the genetic material of the cells, in the production of red blood cells in bone marrow, in the utilization of folic acid and carbohydrates in the diet, and in the functioning of the nervous system.

B_{12}, like other B vitamins, strengthens the immune system. It treats low blood pressure, fights viral infections, and aids in the warding off of asthma and allergy attacks.

All B's work best and are most safe taken together.

The reason? The members of this group—including B_1, B_2, B_3, B_6, folic acid, B_{12}, pantothenic acid, and biotin—all exist together in nature; and every one of them is needed together in your body for them to do what they're supposed to do. In particular, they're needed for energy production and the health of your heart and circulatory system.

B_{12} works with B_6 and folic acid to help prevent heart disease. Folic acid works in the body with B_{12}, so make sure you have enough of both (see *folic acid*

TIPS

A high intake of B_{12} can mask a folic acid deficiency. It's a good idea if you take B_{12} to add folic acid (used by your body to among other things make blood cells, heal wounds, and build muscles) to your supplement list to be sure you are getting enough of it as well.

in this chapter). You might want to take them together to maximize their effectiveness.

Dosage: The RDA is 2 mcg, but as with the RDA of many vitamins, alternative medicine practitioners recommend taking more to treat specific conditions—as much as 100 and 400 mcg. In fact, up to 1 mg per day has been given without side effects as long as the other B vitamins are balanced out and taken with it.

Co-enzyme Q-10

Coenzyme Q10 is found in all living beings and of course is found in the human body. Co-Q10 is a provitamin (which means it allows your body to make a vitamin from it) and is necessary for every cell's storage of energy.

Co-Q10 is like the body's own supply of ginkgo or ginseng. Containing a comprehensive set of all-body health properties, it is already an integral part of your body's systems, with highest concentrations in the heart, liver, kidneys, and pancreas. You can't function without it. Unfortunately, the body often doesn't produce enough Co-Q10 to garner many of its most impressive effects. The good news is that you can take supplements, which can help you function, as a whole, more effectively.

Among the myriad health benefits of Co-Q10 are its actions as an antioxidant in conjunction with vitamin E. Now let me confess: I never quite knew what an antioxidant was, except that it was supposed to protect our bodies from environmental hazards like pollution. Now I know more about the subject, which I'd like to share with you.

Just like it sounds, an antioxidant prevents oxygen from entering our bodies where it's unwelcome. Why would it ever be unwelcome? Because oxygen can actually destroy some substances in our bodies, including vitamins E, A, and C, and it renders some molecules unstable.

Vitamin E and other anti-oxidants "accept" some amounts of oxygen, thereby protecting molecules from it, allowing them to remain strong. In particular, vitamin E protects vitamin A and unsaturated fatty acids from oxidation, and when in the lungs protects cell and red blood cell membranes from pollution and oxidation.

STUDY RESULTS

In a long-term study reported on in the journal *Molecular Aspects of Medicine* 424 patients with various forms of cardiovascular disease had Coenzyme Q10 added to their current medical treatments. The quantity of their dosage ranged anywhere from 75 to 600 mg daily with the average being around 242 mg. After dividing patients up into six diagnostic categories improvements were measured according to the New York Heart Association functional scale and 59 percent improved by at least one category, 28 percent by two, and 1.2 percent by three. Medication requirements overall dropped dramatically with 43 percent of the group stopping between one and three medications.

Mol Aspects Med. 1994;15 Suppl:s165-75.

Usefulness of coenzyme Q10 in clinical cardiology: a long-term study.

Langsjoen H, Langsjoen P, Langsjoen P, Willis R, Folkers K.
University of Texas Medical Branch, Galveston 77551, USA.

Over an eight year period (1985-1993), we treated 424 patients with various forms of cardiovascular disease by adding coenzyme Q10 (CoQ10) to their medical regimens. Doses of CoQ10 ranged from 75 to 600 mg/day by mouth (average 242 mg). Treatment was primarily guided by the patient's clinical response. In many instances, CoQ10 levels were employed with the aim of producing a whole blood level greater than or equal to 2.10 micrograms/ml (average 2.92 micrograms/ml, n = 297). Patients were followed for an average of 17.8 months, with a total accumulation of 632 patient years. Eleven patients were omitted from this study: 10 due to non-compliance and one who experienced nausea. Eighteen deaths occurred during the study period with 10 attributable to cardiac causes. Patients were divided into six diagnostic categories: ischemic cardiomyopathy (ICM), dilated cardiomyopathy (DCM), primary diastolic dysfunction (PDD), hypertension (HTN), mitral valve prolapse (MVP) and valvular heart disease (VHD). For the entire group and for each diagnostic category, we evaluated clinical response according to the New York Heart Association (NYHA) functional scale, and found significant improvement. Of 424 patients, 58 per cent improved by one NYHA class, 28% by two classes and 1.2% by three classes. A statistically significant improvement in myocardial function was documented using the following echocardiographic parameters: left ventricular wall thickness, mitral valve inflow slope and fractional shortening. Before treatment with CoQ10, most patients were taking from one to five cardiac medications. During this study, overall medication requirements dropped considerably: 43% stopped between one and three drugs. Only 6% of the patients required the addition of one drug. No apparent side effects from CoQ10 treatment were noted other than a single case of transient nausea. In conclusion, CoQ10 is a safe and effective adjunctive treatment for a broad range of cardiovascular diseases, producing gratifying clinical responses while easing the medical and financial burden of multidrug therapy.

PMID: 7752828
[PubMed - indexed for MEDLINE]

Back to coenzyme Q10: Co-Q10 has been proven effective in treating heart conditions, including chronic heart failure, congestive heart failure, angina (chest and heart pain), cardiomyopathy, ventricular arrhythmia (an irregular heart beat), and heart surgery. Another plus factor is Co-Q10's ability to stimulate the immune system and trigger energy release in cells. It has been used to help treat high blood pressure, periodontal disease, cancer, and muscular dystrophy.

Coenzyme Q10—sometimes called the "energy enzyme"—promotes mental endurance and stamina. Thought to stave off the effects of aging on the brain by protecting the mitochondria (power centers of the cells), this coenzyme also defends against free radical damage. In research studies, it has significantly extended the life span of test animals.

A 1994 study showed that Co-Q10 taken with vitamin C, vitamin E, beta carotene, selenium, and omega-3 and omega-6 fatty acids effectively halted movement of breast cancer to other organs, and reduced tumor growth in some patients. Another study showed that, combined with iron and vitamin B_6, Co-Q10 minimized symptoms associated with Alzheimer's. Internal absorption of the provitamin is bolstered by our body's supply of B vitamins.

The standard Co-Q10 supplement dosage is 30-60 mg per day. For heart disease, some doctors recommend 100-200 mg per day, and for breast cancer, 90-390 mg per day. Co-Q10 should always be taken with meals that contain some fat; and dosages over 100 mg should be divided throughout the day. If you find a product that says "hydrosoluble," that means it will absorb better, so you may be able to get away with half the regular dosage.

DID YOU KNOW?

In order to keep the testicles around 92 degrees, or six degrees lower than the rest of the body, the scrotal sack will expand or contract.

Warning: A dosage of 100 mg or higher of Co-Q10 taken in the evening may cause mild insomnia. Certain pharmaceutical drugs inhibit the action of Co-Q10; check with your physician.

Copper

Although the only copper coin in circulation today is worth just a penny, copper is a far more valuable—and essential—component to the human body. Its functions include formation of hemoglobin, enzymes, and protein.

Copper is one of the few metallic elements essential to human health. It promotes health in your reproductive system as well as your nervous system, immune system, bones, muscles, connective tissue, hair, and pigmentation. It helps you oxidize vitamin C, absorb iron, inhibit formation of dangerous free radicals, maintain the integrity of cell membranes, lower cholesterol levels, promote formation of neurotransmitters, and protect against cancer. It strengthens blood vessels, promotes blood clotting, and helps maintain fertility.

Zinc interferes with the body's ability to absorb copper. For this reason many experts recommend that if you are taking a zinc supplement for longer than a month you should also supplement with copper.

For thousands of years, copper has been used as a medicine and to purify drinking water—although ironically, some modern filtration systems remove copper from drinking water. Since ancient times, the wearing of copper bracelets has been thought to provide relief for the discomforts of joints and connective tissues including arthritis, rheumatism, inflammation, tendonitis, bursitis, and osteoporosis.

Copper deficiency, which is extremely uncommon, can cause weakness, diarrhea, osteoporosis, emphysema and related respiratory problems, skin sores, and coronary disease. On the other hand, too much copper in the body can cause schizophrenia, heart disease, nausea, vomiting, and abdominal and muscle pain. Excess copper can be removed through chelation or zinc supplementation; popular supplements include copper gluconate and copper sulfate.

Your body can't make copper, so you have to ingest it in your diet or through supplements. Recent studies show that only one in four Americans consumes enough copper to meet the recommended requirements of the US Food and Nutrition Board.

Foods rich in copper include currants, legumes, mushrooms, nuts, raisins, shellfish, whole grains, potatoes, organ meats, black pepper, dark leafy greens, dried fruits, yeast, seeds, chickpeas, artichokes, avocados, radishes, fortified cereals, meat, fish, and cocoa.

Dosage: RDA is 2 mg. The National Research Council estimates the safe and adequate dosage for adults to be 1.5 to 3 mg.

Cordyceps

The process of growth of this substance is fascinating, if not a tad nauseating—also known as caterpillar fungus and winter bug summer herb, this fungus mummifies certain high-altitude insects in their larval stage, completely enclosing them and then growing outward in a stalk from the insect body. The entire fungus and insect body, then, is considered medicinal and is used to treat a wide variety of ailments.

If you can get over the idea of ingesting a mummified bug, cordyceps may help you counteract some of the effects of old age and improve your sexual performance. Used in Chinese medicine for "eternal youth," it is also widely discussed in English medicinal literature, and is primarily known for preventing aging and preventing the deterioration of sexual performance–including treatment for sexual impotence. A 1998 Stanford University review of current research on cordyceps summarizes that proven benefits of the fungus include actions on the endocrine system (that's your entire hormonal shebang) and systems of sexual function.

Cordyceps also benefits the kidneys, lungs, and heart. It aids in gonadal function, and relieves exhaustion and excessive sweating. It has been proven to lower cholesterol, triglycerides, and blood pressure, and to boost the immune system and cell vitalization. Eaten as an ingredient in duck, chicken, pork, or fish stew, cordyceps has been used to treat weakness and debility. It has also been combined with cortex eucommiae ulmoidis, herba epimedii, epimedium, and herba cistanches to treat impotence and effects of weak kidneys. Taken with the seeds of pruni armeniacae, bulbus fritillariae cirrhosae, and gelatinum asini, it can treat cough, wheezing, and chest pain.

This is a supplement that you might need to consult a skilled herbalist or someone trained in traditional Chinese medicine to obtain and have prepared properly.

Dosage: 1 gram of extract twice daily; 209 grams twice daily of the fruiting body.

Caution: Doses of 30 – 50 g per kg of body weight have been shown to be toxic in animals. That's <u>many</u> times in excess of the safe dosage listed above.

DID YOU KNOW?

A human testicle contains around two hundred meters of seminal tubes. If spread from end to end that is more than enough tubing to stretch from one end of a football field to the other.

Cuscutae

We have to thank many host plants for this wonderful herb—the cuscutae plant is a parasite and yields its medicinal seeds only after it has happily inhabited the being of another plant. Maybe it's because it has so much support from friends that the seed can lend so much support to us!

Cuscutae seed is a godsend for many men in their middle and upper years. It addresses many of our most common sex-related ailments, including infertility, impotence, premature ejaculation, symptoms of BPH, and other prostate problems. A 1997 Wannan Medical College (China) study concluded that cuscutae seed increased sperm motility (speed and extent of sperm movement) and supported sperm membrane tissue, making sperm stronger.

Cuscutae has been shown to decrease nocturnal emissions of sperm and to help prevent premature ejaculation, especially when combined with psoralea fruit and eucommia bark. Perhaps most exciting is that cuscutae seed has been proven to reduce certain symptoms of BPH, and even to help treat impotence. Also, cuscutae has also been shown to treat frequent urination, diarrhea, muscular weakness, and dizziness.

Dosage: You can buy the seeds at Chinese or health food stores in bulk, but the appropriate dosage depends on the size and preparation of seeds. I would suggest you rely on the package dosage, the advice of the herbalist where you purchase the seeds, or begin with a very small amount and work your way up, taking account of how your body feels.

Caution: Patients with constipation should not take cuscutae.

Damiana

Damiana is a leaf extract valued as an aphrodisiac by various cultures, including the ancient Mayans. The damiana extract provides beta sitosterol and various aromatic oils that make your body literally tingle with desire—shifting sexual yearning and response into overdrive!

Damiana leaves contain 0.2-1.0% volatile oil, which isn't enough to hurt you, but is enough to stimulate your genitourinary tract. In other words, you'll feel it nicely in your sexual organs. The plant has been used for over a century in the United

States to aid in the cure of impotence and to strengthen the male sexual system.

Almost all sources are quick to report that the aphrodisiac properties of the herb are unproven by empirical western methods. I had a hard time finding any western medical research on this aspect of the substance at all (any researchers out there need a subject?). Yet, the pervasive use of damiana for treatment of sexual dysfunction makes me think there may be some validity in the claims of its effectiveness.

It is also an antidepressant and a strengthener of the central nervous and the hormonal systems and is used in the treatment of respiratory disorders.

As a folk remedy, damiana has been used to induce menstruation in women, treat lung-related problems like asthma, and for relief from coughs, colds, and flu. Combined with oats, it's a soothing nerve tonic. It also combines well with kola or skullcap.

Dosage: 3 to 6 grams daily. Tincture: 1-2 ml 3 times daily.

Warning: Damiana is a stimulant, so avoid taking it at bedtime. It may interfere with hypoglycemic therapy.

Deer Horn

No, this isn't a charming name for an antler-shaped plant; it's actually the ground up antler of a deer. But using ground up animal cartilage as a sexual stimulant is nothing new; powdered rhinoceros horn has long been valued for its aphrodisiac properties. (That's where we get the term "horny.")

The good news for animal lovers is that no deer are killed for their horns. Each spring deer lose their antlers and grow a new set. The old antlers are collected and made into deer antler supplement.

Deer antler has long been regarded as a rejuvenating tonic in folk medicine; the Chinese

Doing the Math

5.08 inches is the average erection length in a study of adult males

3.46 inches is the average flaccid penis length in a study of adult males

3.41 inches is the erection length above which experts would not consider penile augmentation

have known about it for more than 2,000 years. In ancient Rome, wealthy women used a beauty cream containing crushed antlers from healthy young stag mixed into honey. But only recently has western medicine begun to provide clinical evidence of deer antler's ability to increase energy and vitality while building resistance to stress and illness.

For our purposes, it's important to note that deer horn has been used as a home remedy to treat a wide range of male and female sexual disorders. These include impotence, infertility, and menopausal and menstrual disorders. Eastern doctors have used deer antler to treat penile erection dysfunction, enlarged prostate, and watery semen.

Deer antler has also been used to treat many other conditions, ranging from eczema, psoriasis, arthritis, rheumatism, anemia, high blood pressure, kidney disorders, wounds, inflammation, constipation, asthma, liver problems, high cholesterol, and respiratory problems. Other reputed benefits include improved blood production and circulation, liver function, digestion, and the promotion of growth in children.

What makes deer antler so potent? Like shark cartilage, the cartilage in deer antlers contains chondroitin sulfate, a substance that reduces inflammation while inhibiting the enzymes that degrade cartilage cell proteins. Chondroiton sulfate promotes the production and stabilization of connective tissue. It also improves blood circulation and may reduce the risk of heart attack.

The cartilage contains n-acetyl-glucosamine, a substance found to significantly speed up the healing of wounds. Another compound in the cartilage, glycosaminoglycans, regulate the integrity of synovial fluid to keep joints limber and reduce joint stiffness and pain.

In addition to cartilage, the deer antler also contains a broad mix of amino acids, enzymes, minerals, and vitamins. Other components include chondrocytes, chrondroblasts, glycosamine, arginine, male and female hormones, anti-inflammatory prostaglandins, and IGF-1, the insulin growth factor that promotes muscular development.

> **TIPS**
>
> Try morning sex. Your testosterone levels are at their peak in the morning and since you are well rested you may find yourself more in the mood.

DHEA (Dehydroepiandrosterone)

A lot of controversy surrounds this supplement. DHEA is either a miracle anti-aging drug or snake oil, depending on who you're talking to. Dozens of books and articles have been written praising DHEA; and an equal number have been published damning it. So what's the skinny?

To begin with, DHEA is a naturally occurring steroid hormone produced by the adrenal glands. It's a precursor to testosterone, and as you age from 20 to 50, your body's DHEA level drops by 50 percent, By age 90, your level has declined by a total of 90 percent.

Supporters of DHEA say that DHEA modulates diabetes, obesity, carcinogenesis, tumor growth, neurite outgrowth, virus and bacterial infection, stress, hypertension, collagen and skin integrity, fatigue, depression, memory, and immune responses. In some animal studies, DNA extended rodent life spans up to 50 percent.

In a 1994 study at the University of California School of Medicine, middle-age volunteers taking 50 mg DHEA nightly for 3 months reported an increase in physical and psychological well-being. These improvements included enhanced energy, deeper sleep, better mood, more relaxed feelings, and an increased ability to deal with stressful situations.

Side effects: acne and excessive oiliness, irritability or mood change, overstimulation, insomnia, fatigue, low energy, headaches, hair loss, and heart palpitations. Also because DHA is a hormone caution should be exercised by anyone who is at risk for certain types of cancers.

There is no standard DHEA dosage, since some practitioners feel you shouldn't take it at all. Those who favor it recommend anywhere from 25 mg to 100 mg daily for 2 weeks, then 1 week off, then 2 weeks on, and so on. If you take DHEA it is best to start with a very low dose and slowly increase the dosage over time. Consult your doctor before taking DHEA and again 3 months later to test for appropriate DHEA levels in your body.

Dioscoreae (Wild yam)

Some middle-aged or older men may find relief from a number of common and annoying age-related ailments, including frequent urination, inability to urinate, and spermatorrhea (that's the involuntary excretion of ejaculate, not necessarily associated with orgasm). More importantly, it is also thought to nourish the kidneys and lungs, and therefore may be used to ease the affects of some kidney disorders.

Sometimes called Mountain Medicine (which is the literal English translation of the Chinese name Shan Yao), it is also used against diarrhea, fatigue, spontaneous sweating, and lack of appetite. It has been shown to have an anticancer effect in animals, and to exhibit anti-inflammatory activities (remember, anything that's an anti-inflammatory may counteract many kinds of internal and external irritation). Clinical studies have also shown it to lower blood cholesterol.

Unlike many herbs on the market today, wild yam has become an ingredient in a multiplicity of western medicinal drugs. It is reported to be a component of more than 200 million drug prescriptions sold per year, primarily because of its steroidal effects (which means that wild yam enhances the production of hormones, supplying energy to our body's glands and organs so they get what they need to function efficiently).

The first reference to wild yam I've found in folklore was from 25 BCE in China. It has been used as a cure for rheumatism, abdominal pain, gastrointestinal irritation, spasms, and asthma. Native American tribes have also used it as a painkiller.

Daily dosage: 30-60 grains (also for powder and infusion methods). Fluid extract: 2-4 ml. Tincture: 2-10 ml.

NOTE: You might also want to recommend wild yam as an oral supplement for your significant other. A rich source of esterified estrogen compounds, wild yam is recognized by the British Herbal Pharmacopoeia as a treatment to relieve cramps and ovarian and uterine pain.

Epimedium Leaf

My favorite thing about this herb is its common English name: Licentious Goat Wort. The name humorously suggests the most popular application of the leaf, which is to increase sexual activity and sperm production. It stimulates the sensory nerves, thereby increasing sexual desire, and has an androgen-like effect on the testes, prostate gland, and levator ani muscle (that means it acts like a male sex hormone, exciting the sex organs).

Epimedium is used to treat various kidney-related malfunctions, including impotence and frequent urination. It also is said to lower blood pressure, and it is reputed to increase memory. In combination with fructus schisandrae chinensis (schizandra seed), fructus lyci chinensis, and semen astragali (astragalus), epimedium has been used to treat impotence and infertility.

In a study conducted at the Zhejiang Provincial Hospital of Chinese Medicine, epimedium was used to treat 182 men ages 25 to 41 who suffered from low sperm count. In 65 percent of these patients, sperm count increased.

In a separate study conducted at Shanghai People's Hospital, 21 cases of male impotence were treated with an herbal formula containing epimedium. Thirteen of these patients enjoyed a return to normal sexual function within 3 days.

Dosage: 3 – 12 g daily. Possible side effects include dizziness, vomiting, thirst, and nausea.

Eucommia bark

I'll call this one the blood herb, but it also bolsters male sexual capability (by aiding in sperm production) and reduces some effects of aging. You'll find eucommia bark, also called cortex eucommiae and du-zhong leaf, in just 5 percent of the herbal guides you peruse, probably because it seems to be considered viable only within Asian medicinal communities (which means that in five years it will probably be the newly discovered Western thing-of-the-moment!). But numerous Asian studies and references on Chinese medicine point to eucommia bark as beneficial for our blood, our sexual organs, and to reduce the effects of aging.

It's important for men as they age to support their integral blood-related systems. Eucommia has been shown to relieve blood pressure and hypertension. Decoctions of eucommia lower blood pressure and treat hypertension effectively, either actually lowering blood pressure or at least alleviating symptoms of the condition.

Eucommia may also help us with our sex-related organs. It supports the liver and kidneys, and is used to combat frequent urination and infertility in men by increasing the production of sperm. It also aids in circulation (and we all know why we need good circulation) and is used to treat fatigue.

Many recent studies focus on its effects on the stimulation of collagen synthesis, an important anti-aging process (aging inhibits our body's production of collagen, which is a part of your bone, connective tissue, and skin). A 1997 Nihon University (Japan) study shows that used with ginseng, eucommia promotes collagen production and prevents decreased protein metabolism, thereby slowing the effects of aging. According to the study, the most effective combination is one part ginseng to 3 parts eucommia.

Used for medicinal purposes in China for over 3,000 years, this herb is made from the bark of eucommia ulmoides, popularly known as the hardy rubber tree, which can grow to a height of 50 feet. The bark is stripped from the trees, dried in the sun, and crushed to a powder. The glossy leaves, which are 4 to 6 inches long, have more minimal beneficial effects than the bark.

Eucommia has been used as a sedative, tonic, anti-inflammatory, anti-hypertensive, diuretic, diet aid, and back pain treatment. People also take it to tonify liver and kidneys, strengthen bones and tendons, prevent miscarriage, and increase longevity. In Japan, eucommia is a popular sex stimulant. Studies suggest eucommia may help control body fat and cholesterol levels. The tree is not used as a rubber source because it contains very little latex.

Daily dosage: 10 – 15 g. In large doses, it has a mild sedative effect.

Folic acid (folate, folacin)

Folic acid, a B vitamin, has been recommended for years for women who are infertile. There is some evidence now that folic acid can also benefit male potency and sexual function.

Folic acid is a coenzyme for neurotransmitters, chemicals that enable transmission of nerve signals. A deficiency of folic acid therefore can cause depression, negatively effecting mood and sex drive. An article in *Nutrition Reviews* reports that low levels of folic acid have been found in 15 to 38 percent of adults suffering from depression. In one study, 81 percent of depressed elderly patients taking 50 mg daily of methylfolate noticed an improvement.

TIPS

Be sure to supplement with B_{12} if you take a folic acid supplement. Folic acid has the ability to mask a vitamin B_{12} deficiency that can lead to a type of anemia. For this reason there are a number of combination supplements on the market that contain both B_{12} and folic acid.

STUDY RESULTS

According to a recent study published in the journal *Arch Latinoam Nutr* combining B$_{12}$, B$_6$, and folic acid may be an effective way of dropping dangerous homocysteine and cholesterol levels and thus fighting heart disease. Men in the study were given the three supplements daily and their homocysteine, triglycerides, total cholesterol, low-density lipoprotein, and very-low-density lipoprotein all dropped. They also had a slight rise in their good high-density lipoprotein levels.

Arch Latinoam Nutr. 2005 Mar;55(1):28-33.

Effect of the supplementation of vitamins B$_{12}$, B$_6$ and folic acid on homocysteine and plasmatic lipids in patients with hyperlipoproteinemic secondary type IV

Moron de Salim AR, Garces Pasamontes A.

Departamento de Bioquimica, Escuela de Medicina, Facultad de Ciencias de la Salud, Universidad de Carabobo, Valencia, Estado Carabobo, Venezuela.

The cases of hyperlipoproteinemic secondary type IV are manifested by elevation of triglycerides, with normal or high cholesterol and lightly high homocysteine. The effect of vitamins B$_{12}$, B$_6$ and folic acid, on homocysteine and lipids, in 24 male patients, 35-68 years, with hiperlipoproteinemia secondary type IV with myocardial isquemic, and without previous treatment of hipolipemiant, was investigated. The patients were supplemented with therapeutic doses tablets of vitamin B$_{12}$, 500 (microg/day); B$_6$, (600 mg/day) and folic acid (20 mg/ day), during 120 days. Homocysteine, triglycerides, total and fractional cholesterol, at (basal), 30, 60, 90 and 120 days, were determined. Descriptive statistical analyses were applied, coefficient of correlation of Pearson and proves of "t", with a p < 0.005; the data were processed by statistical program SPSS version 8.0. The results showed a decrease in the levels of homocysteine from basal 17.1 +/- 0.7 micromol/L to 13.18 +/- 0.83 micromol/L, at the end of experimental period. The triglycerides (TG), total cholesterol (TC), low density lipoprotein (LDL), very low density lipoprotein (VLDL) showed a reduction of

(21.8 mg/dl; 8.5 mg/dl; 5.87 mg/dl; respectively) for every pmol/L of reduced homocysteine, with (p < 0.001) for triglycerides. High density lipoprotein (HDL) increased 1.1 mg/dl and coronary risk descent in 24%.

> Folic acid can be some over the counter and prescription drugs. Among those that may affect your folic acid levels are:
>
> - aspirin
> - barbiturates
> - corticosteroids
> - NSAIDS
> - choline magnesium and salisylates
> - ranitidine

We concluded that therapeutic doses of vitamins B$_{12}$, B$_6$ and folic acid, may be effective in decreased plasmatic homocysteine levels and lipids, mainly triglycerides, with a reduction of coronary risk, to these type of patients, with not collateral effects of neuropathy.

PMID: 16187675
[PubMed - in process]

As we age, our capacity to absorb sufficient amounts of folic acid from the foods we eat decreases. According to an article in the *New England Journal of Medicine*, four out of ten Americans get too little folic acid in their diet. A sore tongue, apathy, anemia, digestive problems, fatigue, insomnia, paranoia, and memory loss can be indications of folate deficiency.

Folate deficiency can damage the brain and nervous system. In addition, folic acid prevents the undesirable amino acid *homocystine* from building up in the blood. The RDA of 400 mcg folic acid daily lowers homocystine levels by 6 micromol per liter of blood, which reduces risk of circulatory system disease 50 to 80 percent or higher.

Excess levels of homocystine can cause a rare medical condition, Marfan's Syndrome that can produce skeletal deformities. Homocystine build-up also increases your chances of having a heart attack, stroke, coronary heart disease, carotoid artery stenosis, Alzheimer's disease, rectal cancer, and colon cancer.

One study found that men with 15.4 micromol/liter blood homocystine levels had an almost five times greater risk of having a stroke than men with a more normal level of 10.3 micromol/l. In another study, subjects taking 398 mcg of folic acid daily had a 60 percent reduced risk of colorectal adenomas vs. a control group not taking folic acid.

Foods rich in folic acid include leafy dark green vegetables, beans, peas, citrus fruits and juices, whole grains, fortified breakfast cereals, and berries. One study shows that men and women over 60 who take vitamin C tablets had 25 percent more folic acid in their bodies than those who take no vitamin C.

Dosage: 400 mcg daily.

Fo-Ti

Known in China as Ho Shou Wu, this herb is used as a rejuvenating tonic and to promote cardiac health, combat cancer, prevent hair from turning gray, preserve youthfulness, increase energy and vigor, and restore fertility. It is also used as a remedy for insomnia, upset stomach, diabetes, and constipation.

Fo-ti is made from the dried roots of polygonum multiforum, a Chinese evergreen tree. Some researchers suspect that fo-ti may contain compounds with mild anti-inflammatory and cardiovascular compounds—accounting for its believed ability to reduce serum cholesterol levels, incidence of heart disease, and blood pressure. The plant also contains a number of glycosides that may help relieve stomach problems and constipation.

In the Orient Tantric beliefs say that saving sperm increases sexual energy, and ejaculating too frequently depletes sexual energy. Fo-ti is said to inhibit unwanted ejaculations (such as nocturnal emission), savings the energy for sexual intercourse as well as increasing sperm production.

Fo-ti is an ancient herb first recorded in the Tang Dynasty 713 A.D. Its original name was jiaoteng. The herb is not considered a magic bullet treatment and Chinese herbalists will warn you that it is in the slow and moderate group of herbs meaning that to see effects will take time and the effects are not dramatic but rather subtle improvements. Fo-ti users are said to experience good health, vigor, and youth.

Dosage: Fo-ti can be taken as a pill and it is generally recommended that you take a 450 mg supplement 2 to 3 times a day.

Ginkgo Biloba

I was amazed with the research on this one. It turns out that most of the claims we hear from marketing companies touting the miracle effects of ginkgo are supported by western empirical research. Of course, the herb doesn't produce miracles at all; but the variety of beneficial effects ginkgo has is certainly rare in one substance, to say the least.

Whether your ailment is sex-related or not, chances are this ancient tree may be able to help you. If I hadn't already been taking gingko when I did this research, I would have run out and gotten some.

Termed a "living fossil" because this Asian tree species has existed for 200 million years, individual trees can live for as long as 1,000 years! The active ingredients, ginkgo flavone glycosides and terpene lactones, are concentrated in the tree leaves. Ginkgo biloba has been proven in numerous conclusive studies to treat assorted ailments, including sexual dysfunction, memory loss, and circulatory problems.

Gingko biloba increases blood circulation by dilating the airways of the lungs, peripheral blood vessels, arteries and veins. This can have a positive impact on results in almost any blood flow-related disorder. Among those I found most compelling are treatment of impotence and limb debility due to natural age-related reduction of blood flow to the appendages. The herb also has shown some apparent abilities to lower blood pressure, combat depression, aids in hormonal system disorders, treats hemorrhoids, and positively effects the glandular and nervous systems.

For those of us interested in alternatives to Viagra, Levitra or Cialis the best news is that gingko biloba has been shown to increase sexual function. Two decades of research on gingko extract have shown it to have a significant effect on the glandular, cardiovascular, and nervous systems. Gingko helps dilate air passages in the lungs, improve circulation, neutralize dangerous free radicals, increase prostaglandins that control blood pressure, and improve vigor.

A University of California study showed that among subjects who had antidepressant induced sexual dysfunction problems, 91 percent of women and 76 percent of men responded to gingko with an increase in desire, excitement (erection), orgasm, and resolution (afterglow).

And in a study performed by a team of German urologists, 50 men suffering from "arterial erectile impotence" were given 240 mg of ginkgo biloba daily. After 9 months, 78 percent of the men regained the ability to have an erection.

You probably know that one of the most talked about effects of gingko is the reported increase of mental clarity and memory in users. Studies suggest that gingko increases serotonin uptake to the brain—serotonin is the brain chemical that produces our feeling of happiness, and also effects sex drive and energy level. (St. John's Wort and many popular antidepressants, including Prozac, target the management of this chemical, among others). Clinical studies have proven gingko's effectiveness in counteracting what have been thought of as symptoms of normal aging–short term memory loss, headache, ringing in the ears, dizziness, depression, and diabetic impotence.

Numerous studies have shown that ginkgo biloba extract increases blood flow to the microcapillaries of the brain by cleaning out blood vessels, which in turn brings the nutrients your brain needs to function well again. In addition, ginkgo has been shown to increase the speed of neurotransmitter release into the synapses in the brain during mental processes, and to prevent neurotransmitter breakdown by enzymes. This enhances your reflexes, concentration, mental stamina, thought processes, and ability to learn.

Ginkgo biloba enables the brain to consume glucose, its primary fuel, with increased efficiency. It also reduces swelling in the brain common in old age, inhibiting age-related reduction of mental function. That's why it has been called the brain drug—a rare case in which a commercial sales term is actually justified by research!

Studies show that ginkgo may increase alpha rhythms, which are the brain waves associated with creativity, relaxation, and healing. Alpha brain activity is also associated with what is known as "super learning"—the ability to learn, process, store, and recall large amounts of information quickly and efficiently. According to a study published in the *Journal of the American Medical Association*, a U.S. study of patients with mild to moderate dementia showed that those who took gingko scored higher on mental performance tests than a control group taking a placebo. According to a review published in 2004 in the German journal *Current Pharmaceutical Design*.

"[Ginkgo biloba] may be a tremendously important compound for slowing the progression of neurodegenerative disorders like Alzheimer's disease," reports the chief of the pharmacological treatment research program at the National Institute of Mental Health.

Adds Dr. Turan Itil, chairman of the New York Institute for Medical Research, "The more than 100 memory-clinic patients I work with who have been taking ginkgo for over 2 years are satisfied with the treatment."

> The gingko leaf when it has not been processed is capable of producing severe allergic reactions. Never use the unprocessed leaves in any form. Stick to standardized extracts in which the allergens have been safely removed.

Gingko biloba has been used medicinally in China since at least 1350 BC. Given the myriad of positive effects of the herb, it is no wonder that it is believed to lengthen the life span, according to Chinese and Western folklore. But I found it most unusual that it is also widely believed to clear up air pollution wherever it is planted (and thrives in its own clean air in filthy urban centers across the world). It is resistant to pollution, virus, and fungi. Maybe we should be buying gingko biloba trees along with our electric cars!

So it's probably obvious why gingko is one of my favorites. It's likely to help sexual dysfunction. But even if you're one of the few for whom it doesn't work in this capacity, chances are it will help you in numerous other ways.

Dosage: Standard dosage is 120 mg daily, 40 mg three times, but studies have been conducted from 40-600 mg daily.

Side effects (rare): stomach or intestinal upset or headaches.

Ginseng (panax ginseng)

If you were around in the 70's, chances are you knew people who started visiting the then small and locally owned organic health food stores and touting the multiple and diverse benefits of this "new" panacea. Hardly new, ginseng is an ancient Asian remedy that has been used for centuries to treat an amazing variety of ailments. And luckily for us, the substance is now easy to find.

Like ginkgo, ginseng promises to assist those of us in our middle years (or as I like to think of it, my "late youth") with many of our most common ailments. It is used to fight impotence and increase sexual appetite and vitality; to increase learning and memory capacity, work performance, and life span; to counteract the natural aging process; and to enhance the body's immune system. It has also been used to treat cancer, diabetes, hypotension, fatigue, stress, asthma, depression, anxiety, and heart disease.

But don't run out and buy everything that says "ginseng" (you may have noticed that these days everything, from tea to chocolate, comes with added ginseng to rope in the health conscious consumer). The problem is, not all ginseng is made alike. Two of the primary elements of ginseng are the saponin groups Rg1 and Rb1. Types of ginseng vary according to the ratio of these conflicting ingredients, which combine to achieve a more or less beneficial balance.

> **M**ake sure you are getting panax ginseng (also called Asian, Chinese, or Korean ginseng). Other kinds of ginseng, like American or Siberian, have different effects on the body.

You probably want Chinese ginseng (Rg1-dominant), in the water soluble form, if your concerns (like mine) are sexual function, brain power, or fatigue. The best form of this type of ginseng is wild mountain root or "Ye Shan Shen." Chinese ginseng also aids the respiratory system, combats excessive urination, reduces blood sugar levels, lowers cholesterol, aids in protein synthesis, and increases appetite.

CAUTION!

If you are taking any MAO inhibitor drugs, have any heart rhythm irregularities, or uncontrollable high blood pressure do not take ginseng.

American Ginseng (Rb1-dominant) will also give your vital organs a little stimulation and reportedly will relieve fatigue, but it isn't nearly as beneficial as Chinese.

In one double-blind study reported on in the *The Journal of Urology* scientists tested the effects of Korean red ginseng on a group of patients with clin-

STUDY RESULTS

If you are diabetic you may benefit from ginseng. Several studies have shown that ginseng can potentially lower blood sugar levels in diabetics. Interestingly one study, published in the journal *Phytomedicine* found that while both ginseng root and ginseng berries appear to have the ability to lower blood sugar levels the berries appear to also have the ability to reduce body weight.

Phytomedicine. 2003;10(6-7):600-5.

Anti-hyperglycemic effects of ginseng: comparison between root and berry.

Dey L, Xie JT, Wang A, Wu J, Maleckar SA, Yuan CS.
Tang Center for Herbal Medicine Research, Chicago, Illinois, USA.

Previous studies demonstrated that both ginseng root and ginseng berry possess anti-diabetic activity. However, a direct comparison between the root and the berry under the same experimental conditions has not been conducted. In the present study, we compared anti-hyperglycemic effect between Panax ginseng root and Panax ginseng berry in ob/ob mice, which exhibit profound obesity and hyperglycemia that phenotypically resemble human type-2 diabetes. We observed that ob/ob mice had high baseline glucose levels (195 mg/dl). Ginseng root extract (150 mg/kg body wt.) and ginseng berry extract (150 mg/kg body wt.) significantly decreased fasting blood glucose to 143 +/- 9.3 mg/dl and 150 +/- 9.5 mg/dl on day 5, respectively (both P < 0.01 compared with the vehicle). On day 12, although fasting blood glucose level did not continue to decrease in the root group (155 +/- 12.7 mg/dl), the berry group became normoglycemic (129 +/- 7.3 mg/dl; P < 0.01). We further evaluated glucose tolerance using the intraperitoneal glucose tolerance test. On day 0, basal hyperglycemia was exacerbated by intraperitoneal glucose load, and failed to return to baseline after 120 min. After 12 days of treatment with ginseng root extract (150 mg/kg body wt.), the area under the curve (AUC) showed some decrease (9.6%). However, after 12 days of treatment with ginseng berry extract (150 mg/kg body wt.), overall glucose exposure improved significantly, and the AUC decreased 31.0% (P < 0.01). In addition, we observed that body weight did not change significantly after ginseng root extract (150 mg/kg body wt.) treatment, but the same concentration of ginseng berry extract significantly decreased body weight (P < 0.01). These data suggest that, compared to ginseng root, ginseng berry exhibits more potent anti-hyperglycemic activity, and only ginseng berry shows marked anti-obesity effects in ob/ob mice.

PMID: 13678250
[PubMed - indexed for MEDLINE]

ically diagnosed erecticle dysfunction. The patients taking the ginseng had significantly higher erectile function scores than those treated with a placebo. Penetration and maintenance of erections were significantly higher in the ginseng group as well. Scans of the penile tips of the ginseng group showed significant improvement in rigidity over the placebo group. The researchers concluded that Korean red ginseng is an affective alternative for treating male erectile dysfunction.

In Asia, ginseng is reputed to extend the life span, which makes sense given its variety of vital beneficial effects. It is included in the medicinal records of various Native American tribes, having been used for centuries by many peoples in the Northeast United States to treat a multiplicity of ailments.

Dosage: 200 mg a day. If using dry root ginseng in the tea or chewable forms some experts recommend 0.5 to 2 g of dry root per day on a short-term basis 1-9 grams. (Remember, wild mountain roots are considered the best, but are the most expensive.)

Side Effects: Although ginseng is considered a safe well tolerated herbal, some rare side effects can occur such as nausea, diarrhea, euphoria, insomnia, headaches, and blood pressure abnormalities

Cautions: Caution should be used if you are already taking phenelzine (Nardil), warfarin (Coumadin), oral hypoglycemics, insulin, or caffeine, or if you have hypertension or bleeding

Glycine

Remember from chapter 1 that your prostate is filled with fluids? Glycine, an amino acid, is one of those fluids—and evidence suggests it may be useful in maintaining prostate health. In one study, 45 men with BPH took approximately 400 mg glycine daily. After 2 months, the men experienced reduced BPH symptoms. Other studies on the role of glycine on BPH symptoms used dosages from 390 mg to 780 mg a day.

Glycine is an important building block of collagen the main protein in connective tissues in the body. Collagen is the main component of ligaments and tendons and it is responsible for skin elasticity.

Glycine also functions as an inhibitory neural transmitter in the central nervous system, meaning that excess glycine may be able to stop unwanted nerve impulses.

In a study published in the Archives of General Psychiatry, schizophrenia patients taking glycine along with the regular antipsychotic medicine showed a 30 percent improvement in symptoms compared with a control group taking the antipsychotic medicine only. Other studies show glycine to be effective in treating chronic spasms, multiple sclerosis, epileptic seizures, and manic psychological states.

Your body makes glycine in the liver and kidneys from choline and amino acids. That's fortunate, since your body has a lot of other uses for glycine aside from improving mood and taking care of your prostate. For instance, glycine is needed to make hemoglobin, the molecule that transports oxygen in your blood. It can also help reduce gastric acidity, stimulate growth, heal wounds, combat free radicals, cleanse the liver, increase glucose available for energy, enhance RNA and DNA production, and boost your immune system. Phew!

Good sources of glycine include fish, meat, beans, dairy, and other foods rich in protein.

Caution: If you have kidney or liver disease, consult your doctor before taking glycine or any other amino acid.

DID YOU KNOW ?

On the 15th of March every year in the Japanese town of Komako a big festival is thrown to celebrate the penis and fertility. A 900 pound wooden phallus is hoisted up and paraded around the streets and women join in the celebration by carrying huge phalluses around in their arms.

Gotu Kola (Hydrocotyle)

Gotu Kola has quite the romantic reputation, due to its age-old use in Asian cultures as a general panacea. It is thought to bolster the immune system, increase longevity, build connective tissues, strengthen veins, and most recently, to support the genito-urinary tract, the last of which is certainly the most exciting to us.

Gotu Kola affects our sexual system because it supports and stimulates the nervous system (see the explanation of the connection between the nervous system and erection in chapter 1). For the same reason, it aids in our brain function, including clarity of thought and memory.

Gotu kola is called by a number of other names including Indian pennywort, Indian water navelwort, talepetrako, Centella asiatica, and hydrocotyle.

In numerous cultures, Gotu Kola is used to heal wounds and as a skin treatment, primarily because of its

STUDY RESULTS

An animal study, published in *Clin Exp Pharmacol Physiol* found that gotu kola positively effected thought processes, increasing cognitive behavior. In addition the substance was found to be an antioxidant combating the oxidative stress that is associated with Alzheimer's disease and cognitive deficits. Other animal studies have had similar results.

Clin Exp Pharmacol Physiol. 2003 May-Jun;30(5-6):336-42.

Effect of Centella asiatica on cognition and oxidative stress in an intracerebroventricular streptozotocin model of Alzheimer's disease in rats.

Veerendra Kumar MH, Gupta YK.

Neuropharmacology Laboratory, Department of Pharmacology, All India Institute of Medical Sciences, Ansari Nagar, New Delhi, India.

1. Centella asiatica, an Indian medicinal plant, has been described as possessing central nervous system activity, such as improving intelligence. In addition, we have demonstrated that C. asiatica has cognitive-enhancing and anti-oxidant properties in normal rats. Oxidative stress or an impaired endogenous anti-oxidant mechanism is an important factor that has been implicated in Alzheimer's disease (AD) and cognitive deficits seen in the elderly.

2. Intracerebroventricular (i.c.v.) streptozotocin (STZ) in rats has been likened to sporadic AD in humans and the cognitive impairment is associated with free radical generation in this model. Therefore, in the present study, the effect of an aqueous extract of C. asiatica (100, 200 and 300 mg/kg for 21 days) was evaluated in i.c.v. STZ-induced cognitive impairment and oxidative stress in rats.

3. Male Wistar rats were injected with STZ (3 mg/kg, i.c.v.) bilaterally on the days 1 and 3. Cognitive behaviour was assessed using passive avoidance and elevated plus-maze paradigms on the days 13, 14 and 21. Rats were killed on the day 21 for estimation of oxidative stress parameters (malondialdehyde (MDA), glutathione, superoxide dismutase and catalase) in the whole brain upon completion of the behavioural task.

4. Rats treated with C. asiatica showed a dose-dependent increase in cognitive behaviour in both paradigms. A significant decrease in MDA and an increase in glutathione and catalase levels were observed only in rats treated with 200 and 300 mg/kg C. asiatica. 5. The present findings indicate that an aqueous extract of C. asiatica is effective in preventing the cognitive deficits, as well as the oxidative stress, caused by i.c.v. STZ in rats.

PMID: 12859423
[PubMed - indexed for MEDLINE]

STUDY RESULTS

Pharmacol Biochem Behav. 2003 Feb;74(3):579-85.

Effect of Centella asiatica on pentylenete-trazole-induced kindling, cognition and oxidative stress in rats.

Gupta YK, Veerendra Kumar MH, Srivastava AK.
Neuropharmacology Laboratory, Department of Pharmacology, All India Institute of Medical Sciences, Ansari Nagar, 110029, New Delhi, India.

Cognitive impairment in epileptics may be a consequence of the epileptogenic process as well as antiepileptic medication. Thus, there is a need for drugs, which can suppress epileptogenesis as well as prevent cognitive impairment. In the present study, the effect of aqueous extract of Centella asiatica (CA) (100 and 300 mg/kg), an Indian medicinal plant known to possess antiepileptic, cognitive-enhancing and antioxidant property, was evaluated on the course of kindling development, kindling-induced learning deficit and oxidative stress markers in pentylenetetrazole (PTZ) kindled rats. Male Wistar rats were injected PTZ (30 mg/kg ip) once every alternate day (48+/-2 h) until the development of the kindling. Passive avoidance test and spontaneous locomotor activity were carried out 24 and 48 h after the last administration of PTZ, while the oxidative stress parameters (malondialdehyde [MDA] and glutathione) were carried out in the whole brain upon completion of the behavioral assessment. The administration of CA (300 mg/kg orally) decreased the PTZ-kindled seizures and showed improvement in the learning deficit induced by PTZ kindling as evidenced by decreased seizure score and increased latencies in passive avoidance behavior. However, low dose of the CA (100 mg/kg) showed improvement only in the learning deficit due to the kindling and failed to improve the seizure score. The findings suggest the potential of aqueous extract of CA as adjuvant to antiepileptic drugs with an added advantage of preventing cognitive impairment.

PMID: 12543222
[PubMed - indexed for MEDLINE]

components of essential oil, saponins, polysaccharides, flavonoids, and glycoside asiaticoside, all of which have been shown to heal.

Dosage: 200 mg liquid extract or 400-500 mg of the crude herb three times a day. There are also various patented brand-name products, including Centasium, Centelase, Emdecassol, and Madecassol that are to be taken in various dosages, as indicated by their manufacturers.

Side effects/precautions: No side effects or toxicity have been shown with the proper dosage, but rare side effects do exist. Headache, skin rash, and sensitivity to sunlight may develop in rare cases. High doses may result in nausea.

Those allergic to propylene glycol should not take it in large amounts. Do not take it if you are engaged in hypoglycemic therapy. It may raise serum-cholesterol levels.

Green Tea

They say you <u>can</u> have too much of a good thing, which is why caffeine's gotten a bad rap. Because the fact is, in reasonable doses like the amount found in many green teas, it has beneficial properties, particularly if what you're looking for is stimulation (aren't we all?).

For more reasons than their caffeine content, green and black teas have been used in China and Japan for centuries to treat a wide variety of ailments. Green tea in particular has been proven to have cancer-fighting properties. One Saitama Cancer Center Research Institute (Japan) study demonstrated that green tea inhibited the growth of cancerous cells in the skin, stomach, duodenum (a section of the small intestine), colon, liver, lung, and pancreas. (The study, though, was based on consumption of ten-plus cups of green tea per day over a number of years—did the drinkers ever have time for anything else?) Green and black teas have also been shown to combat diarrhea, act as diuretics, and to increase mental clarity.

The active ingredient in green tea, which provides protection against illness, is a class of compounds called catechins. These polyphenolic antioxidants, a sub-group of flavonoids, give green tea a higher antioxidant content than either grape juice or red wine. Current research suggests that catechins are at least 25 times more potent than vitamin E and 100 times more potent than vitamin C.

So what does this have to do with your sex life? As a general stimulant, green tea increases blood flow to certain areas of the body (including those of a sexual nature). It has also been shown to possibly inhibit some common diseases or disorders that are likely to prevent a healthy sex life. And, two Saitama (Japan) studies showed that green tea protected against disorders of the liver and colon, respectively. As a

TABLE 4

Caffeine Content of Several Popular Drinks

Drink	Caffeine Content
Vivarin	200 mg
Coffee (8 oz brewed.)	80 - 135 mg
Jolt Cola (12 oz)	71.2 mg
Tea (8 oz brewed.)	30 - 70 mg
Coca-Cola Classic (12 oz)	34 mg
Green tea (8 oz.)	15 mg
Chocolate milk (6 oz.)	8 mg
Decaf coffee (8 oz brewed.)	3 - 4 mg

powerful antioxidant green tea may fight the oxidative stress that can lead to erectile dysfunction.

Black and green teas have been used in the United States to wash tired eyes, to treat skin breakouts, for morning sickness, and for headaches. Green tea is also used as a kidney stimulant, and has been marketed as a slimming agent (its ability to help people lose weight has not been verified by studies). The high antioxidant content of green teas make them likely heart disease and cancer fighting candidates. The teas antimicrobial properties have been shown to suppress the growth of some bacteria including E. coli. and staphylococcus.

Dosage: To prevent oxidation of the catechins, green tea is made from fresh, unfermented tea leaves. The standard dilution is one teaspoon per cup of hot water, but the importance lies in the steeping time. Contrary to popular belief, the longer you let it steep, the less caffeine you'll consume (one account says that's because the caffeine actually dissolves in the hot water). So if you let it steep for two minutes, the stimulant effects will be strongest. Let it go for ten and it will treat your diarrhea.

Green tea is also available in supplements. If using a supplement make sure it is standardized to contain at least 50% polyphenols. If choosing to drink the delicious tea instead four cups of freshly brewed tea will supply the recommended amount of polyphenols.

Combinations: Milk reduces the possible deleterious effects of high tannin levels in tea. It will also make it taste better. The use of tea with muffins has been proven to increase happiness in children and middle age men.

Caution: Consuming green tea in large amounts may contribute to cancer of the esophagus. However, adding milk is thought to bind the tannins in the tea, counteracting any negative effects. In addition avoid drinking the tea to hot which can lead to damage to the throat and esophagus over time increasing your cancer risks. Instead enjoy your tea warm, but not boiling, like it is served in Asia.

Horny Goat Weed (Barrenwort)

You have to love any herb with the name Horny Goat Weed and this one definitely doesn't disappoint. It's use as a medicinal herb dates back centuries. In traditional Chinese medicine barrenwort is typically used to treat kidney problems, impotence, premature ejaculation, and as an aphrodisiac. This low-growing herb is native to the more temperate regions of Europe and Asia.

The herb has been shown to dilate blood vessels and raise dopamine levels. This rise in dopamine levels may be the key to the weed's reported ability to help with impotence issues and aid in male virility. Increased dopamine levels can lead to the release of testosterone.

Dosage: Barrenwort comes in capsules, tablets, powders, and teas. The recommended dosage is usually 1000 to 3000 mg a day. It is recommended for short term use.

Side Effects: No serious side effects have been reported but some users may experience dizziness, dry mouth, or increased sweating.

Inosine

A lady of the evening approached a middle aged man and said, "I'll do anything you want for fifty dollars." His reply: "Paint my garage."

One reason many men have infrequent or no sex is a lack of vitality: They are simply too tired to want it, much less get it up. If you agree that sex is at least partly an athletic exercise requiring stamina and endurance, you can take a tip from athletes and do what they do to increase their energy: take inosine.

A purine nucleotide, inosine (hypoxanthine riboside) is a metabolic activator that increases your body's ability to handle physical activity. Inosine easily penetrates cardiac and skeletal muscle cells to generate ATP (adenosine triphosphate), a vital substance that enhances respiration and oxygen transport as well as muscle contractions during sex, exercise, sports, and other exertion. Inosine promotes the synthesis of 2, 3 diphosphog lyceate, a substance that enables oxygen to be transported from the blood to the muscles.

Other functions of inosine include anti-inflammatory actions, insulin release, use of carbohydrates by heart tissue, and contractions of the heart muscle. Inosine has been used to treat myocarditis, myocardiosclerosis, cardiac arrhythmia, and heart attack.

DID YOU KNOW

The word testicle derives from the Latin word testis meaning witness. The testes are witnesses to a man's virility. There is no truth to the folklore that in ancient Rome men giving an oath would cup their testicles giving rise to the words testify, testimonial, and testament.

Foods rich in inosine include Brewer's yeast and organ meats, such as liver and kidneys.

Irish Moss (Chondrus crispus)

Irish moss is a seawood found in the Atlantic coast of Europe and North America. The extract of the seawood, known as carrageenan, is often used as thickener or stabilizer in processed foods such as ice cream and lunchmeat.

Traditionally the water plant has been used to treat respiratory illnesses, digestive complaints and urinary inflammations. It's the plants possible use to treat urinary inflammations that earned it a spot on our A to Z list. The herb has been shown to have anti-viral, anti-inflammatory and anti-coagulant properties in recent animal research.

Dosage: Steep half an ounce of the dried herb in cold water for 15 minutes and then boil for 10-15 minutes in 3 pints of water (or milk). Strain liquid and add lemon, ginger, or cinnamon, and/or sweetener to taste.

The herb is also available in capsule form. Two 580 mg capsules twice a day with meals is recommended.

Cautions: Because Irish Moss has some blood thinning properties those on anti-coagulant medications should avoid the herb.

Kelp

Kelp is a brown algae, or seaweed, that grows in ocean water. Western studies are just beginning to show the beneficial effects kelp can have, but you might want to trust the centuries of experience of Asian peoples on this one. Used extensively in Asian cultures for both food and remedy for centuries, kelp is still among the herbs in the process of testing for western medical use. But the apparent multiple beneficial effects of it may be worth consideration even before extensive research is completed.

According to Asian studies and current western studies in Japanese communities where kelp is consumed regularly, kelp may fight impotence and infertility, reduce the size of the prostate, and treat uterine disorders and kidney problems.

An early article in the *Asian Medical Journal* stated that clinical studies have shown that daily kelp consumption by older men with enlarged prostate glands gradually reduces the size of the prostate and renders urination painless.

Kelp is mysterious. No one seems to know why it affects the body the way it does, but it has been speculated that it has something to do with the trace minerals contained in the herb, which are essential to gland and organ hormone regulation.

In Japan, where kelp is an integral part of the diet, cases of breast cancer, heart disease, respiratory disease, rheumatism and arthritis, high blood pressure, thyroid deficiency, and gastro-intestinal ailments are very few. Studies show that in Japanese societies where the consumption of kelp has been lowered for various reasons, the cases of all of these diseases and ailments have risen.

Kelp, which is rich in iodine, is also used as a diet drug for reducing fat, because it helps stimulate the thyroid gland. This optimizes your metabolism, enabling your body to burn fat faster so you lose weight. Kelp's effectiveness as a diet supplement, however, has not been proven.

Kelp is also known as an anti-bacterial agent, to cleanse the blood, and to boost the immune system. Other names for kelp include: seaweed, black tang, bladderwrack, kelpware, rockweed, and seawrack.

Much of the above information is considered folklore by the Western medical community, since an extensive body of Western research is still unavailable. However, at the very least kelp is a nutritious food packed with cartenoids, proteins and minerals. You can add kelp to your diet by eating more Asian dishes or try a supplement.

Dosage: Dried kelp, 5 – 10 g three times daily. Liquid extract (one part kelp, one part water in 25% alcohol): 4 – 8 ml three times daily.

Note: Kelp's iodine content may cause hyper or hypothyroidism, as well as aggravate pre-existing acne conditions, at doses exceeding 150 mcg iodine per day.

L-arginine (arginine)

I really can't say enough about this amino acid, especially if we're discussing loss of erection, or recovery thereof.

One of the greatest things about l-arginine is that it works with the natural substances and processes of the male body to perform its beneficial functions. L-arginine has been proven as effective as many prescription drugs for impotence or infertility, but doesn't add any substances to the body that don't already exist there naturally. I don't know about you but I feel better taking stuff that I know is already part of my body.

Studies abound about the beneficial effects of l-arginine on male sexual and reproductive activity, suggesting that it is perhaps the most effective substance for restoring male sexual potency. It does this by increasing the amount of nitric oxide—an odorless gas made of nitrogen and oxygen—into your system.

Nitric oxide is absolutely necessary for erections. If you don't have enough of it, you probably can't get it up, or at least can't keep it there. And if that's your only deficiency, how lucky you are that it may can take one simple supplement to solve your problems! (That sounds like I'm being flippant, but for many men it really is that simple.)

Nitric oxide is vital to achieving and maintaining an erection. Men with insufficient nitric oxide in the bloodstream may suffer from soft, limp erections or even may be unable to get an erection altogether.

Numerous clinical studies have demonstrated nitric oxide's ability to help men create and maintain a stiff erection for a prolonged period. A study published in the *Journal of Urology* concludes: "Nitric oxide is the principle mediator of erectile function." In fact, the 1998 Nobel Prize for Medicine was awarded to three American scientists for their investigation into the properties of nitric oxide.

How does l-arginine increase your body's supply of nitric oxide? Arginine is a rich source of nitrogen, supplying nitrogen atoms to the body. It acts as a vehicle for transport, storage, and excretion of nitrogen. The body combines the nitrogen molecules from the l-arginine with oxygen in the bloodstream to create nitric oxide.

One study conducted at Tel Aviv University demonstrated the powerful impotence fighting potential of l-arginine. After six weeks of taking the supplement 31% of the men who were suffering with impotence had improved versus a 9% improvement with a placebo. (On an interesting side-note the placebo effect makes a strong argument for the power of mind over matter. A positive attitude can go a long way towards overcoming impotence issues.)

Nitric oxide is found naturally in the body inside the epithelial cells that line the blood vessels. When these cells are stimulated, they release nitric oxide, relaxing your muscles and increasing blood flow. In an Oxford Radcliffe Hospital study, researchers showed that l-arginine achieves relaxation of longitudinal layers of human smooth muscle, leading to immediate synthesis and release of nitric oxide. This action increases blood flow to the penis, resulting in erections that are bigger, harder, and more frequent.

During an erection, blood flow equivalent to ten times the normal supply rapidly enters the penis, filling several channels. When the outer walls of the engorged veins are pushed outward, they shut off these channels, preventing the blood from leaving the penis and the man from losing his erection.

In a joint study performed by Dr. Adrian Zargniotti of the New York University School of Medicine and Dr. Eli F. Lizza of the University of Medicine and Dentistry of New Jersey, 15 men under age 65 with a long-standing inability to have erections were treated with 1400 mg of l-arginine daily for 2 weeks. Six of the men reported a "marked improvement" in their ability to perform sexually with harder and longer-lasting erections. In another study, researchers at the John Hopkins University Department of Urology gave men shots of inhibitors designed to prevent erection. Dosages of l-arginine wiped out the inhibitor's negative effects, enabling the men to become erect.

In addition to enabling men who were previously dysfunctional to become erect, l-arginine gives men greater staying power and intensity, while increasing sperm production. It also increases libido, which is the desire for sex, in both men *and* women.

CAUTION!

A special note for herpes sufferers. There have been some anecdotal report of l-arginine stimulating the herpes virus and although this theory is unproven you might want to avoid this supplement to avoid possible flare-ups.

Better sex is not the only benefit of increasing arginine in your system. Nitric oxide offers numerous other benefits to your system. It reportedly may help control blood pressure, boost your immune function, kill microorganisms and cancer cells, and help control muscular activity, balance, and coordination.

A review of the medical literature shows ample evidence that l-arginine stimulates the release of growth hormone, making it critical to the human growth process. It also increases collagen in the body (collagen is the main supportive fibrous protein found in bone, cartilage, and other connective tissue), which in turn enables both protein synthesis and tissue repair.

There is evidence that l-arginine helps stimulate the immune system overall, combats mental and physical fatigue, and helps build muscle mass while decreasing body fat.

L-arginine has long been used in the treatment of hepatic disorders—diseases of the liver. The nitrogen in the l-arginine helps detoxify ammonia, which is poisonous to living cells.

So, how can you get more l-arginine in your diet? Meat, dairy products, poultry, beans, and fish are rich in the substance.

Dosage: L-arginine is also available as a supplement in caplet, tablet, and powder form. The recommended daily dosage of l-arginine for men looking to reverse inadequate erection is approximately 1,000 to 2,000 mg.

L-Carnitine (Carnitine)

L-Carnitine is a vitamin-like compound that is helpful in fighting many diseases and maintaining normal heart function. It is essential for energy production and for fat metabolism. Carnitine is stored in abundance in a well-functioning heart so it can provide energy to the heart when oxygen supply is limited, as with angina and other cardiovascular problems.

Because of its role in energy metabolism, turning fat into energy, L-Carnitine is traditionally used to support any body functions that have a high-energy demand. Like, for example, a really good romp in the sack.

L-Carnitine is present in the foods we eat, but is found in higher concentrations in food of animal origin. The highest levels can be found in lamb, venison, and beef.

The human body stores about 20 grams of L-Carnitine in skeletal muscles, the liver, and heart. Any remaining in the system is excreted in the urine and must be replaced by the synthesis of the substance in the body (about 10% of your needs), diet, and supplementation.

L-Carnitine plays an important role in male fertility. There is a high concentration of the substance in sperm, which is used in energy metabolism and many experts believe in addition supports the sperm quality. L-Carnitine supplementation in infertile men was found to increase sperm count, concentration, and motility.

L-Carnitine might be valuable in maintaining a healthy heart as well. Since the heart obtains 70% of its energy from fat breakdown the role that L-Carnitine plays in turning fat into energy makes it a crucial energy source for the heart.

Lotus seeds
(semen nelumbo nucifera or water lily seeds)

Notice the use of the word "semen" in the scientific name of this herb. "Semen" means "seed" when used in a plant name; *semen nelumbo nucifera* is the seed of the lotus flower.

In Asian folklore, the lotus is a fertility symbol; the belief is that the more seeds there are in a given plant, the more sons you'll have! As a folk remedy, lotus seed has been used to nourish the blood, tranquilize the mind, reinforce the kidneys, tonify the spleen, and treat diarrhea, constipation, palpitations, irritability, and insomnia.

DID YOU KNOW

Some people actually suffer from a phobia, ithyphallophobia, that makes them fear thinking about, seeing or having an erect penis.

Dosage: The seeds can be candied or used in sauces and fillings, desserts, and soups. As a supplement it is recommended you take 25 mg daily.

Lysine

Lysine is one of a number of amino acids your body needs for tissue repair and growth. However your body cannot manufacture its own lysine. You must get it from an outside source. Lysine plays an important role in the production of certain enzymes, hormones, and antibodies that fight off disease.

Research has shown that lysine can inhibit the growth of the herpes simplex virus (HSV). It does this by competing with arginine (another amino acid HSV needs to grow) for absorption into tissue cells. By restricting arginine in your diet and increasing lysine you can manage HSV infections reducing the number and severity of outbreaks. Approximately four out of five patients studied said taking 1–2 grams daily helped reduce herpes outbreaks and symptoms. In addition, lysine maintains nitrogen balance, essential to formation of NO, the nitrogen-oxygen compound that stimulates male erection.

Lysine may help reduce angina pectoris, the chest pain caused by insufficient oxygen in the heart muscle. Lysine stops viral growth and reproduction, gets rid of mouth blisters and cold sores, and enhances production of hormones, enzymes, and antibodies. Research is conflicting on whether or not it can lower or raise serum triglyceride levels so its best for those who have any cholesterol issues or cardiovascular problems to check with their health care provider before increasing their lysine intake.

Lysine helps the body absorb calcium and plays a key role in the formation of collagen, the material from which connective tissue, skin, cartilage, and bone are built. Therefore, it can aid in recovery from injury and surgery.

Since your body cannot produce lysine it must come from foods or supplements. A deficiency of lysine can result in inadequate immune function, loss of energy, bloodshot eyes, irritability, hair loss, anemia, and increased risk of kidney stones. Foods rich in lysine include lean meats, fish, potatoes, cheese, milk, yeast, eggs, fruits, vegetables, chicken, bean sprouts, and beans. However lysine is particularly sensitive to food processing and foods may lose some of their lysine punch if roasted or toasted. For this reason in this case supplements may be a useful alternative.

Dosage: 12 mg lysine per kilogram (2.2 lbs.) of body weight. For a person weighing 145 lbs., the daily dosage would be approximately 2 g.

Magnesium

Man and all other animals on some level depend on plants for their very survival. Without magnesium, plants–and therefore animals and man–would not exist. It is the single magnesium atom in the chlorophyll molecule that enables plants to convert the energy from sunlight into food. In humans, magnesium activates enzymes necessary for neuromuscular contraction, cardiac function, and regulation of the acid-base balance in the body.

Magnesium is a very active element. If you light a strip of pure magnesium with a Bunsen burner in a laboratory, it will burn with an intensely bright, white flame.

Biologically, magnesium acts as a sort of catalyst, helping the body use many nutrients more efficiently. These include carbohydrates, amino acids, fats, calcium, phosphorous, sodium, potassium, and vitamins B, C, and E. Magnesium also promotes the synthesis of nucleic acids and proteins.

Magnesium is needed for the formation of bone,

> **M**agnesium citrate is the form most easily absorbed by the body. There are also magnesium oxide supplements available. However although the oxide form is less costly it is poorly absorbed by the body.

protein, and fatty acids. It assists in making new cells, activates B vitamins, helps blood clot, and is part of the process that allows insulin to be secreted.

Foods rich in magnesium include milk, cheese, meat, seafood, nuts, blackstrap molasses, soybeans, seeds, wheat germ, oatmeal, cornmeal, and rice. Processed foods lose much of their magnesium during processing. Boiling or simmering food in water also depletes the magnesium content.

> **CAUTION!**
>
> If you suffer from kidney disease or are taking tetracycline antibiotics be sure to consult with your doctor before taking a magnesium supplement.

Experts suspect magnesium deficiency as being a cause of a whole host of health problems. These include muscle spasms, tremors, convulsions, depression, sleep disturbances, high blood pressure, vision problems, stress, and increased risk of heart disease.

Dosage: Magnesium is most easily absorbed by the body when taken in aspartate or citrate forms. The RDA for men is 400 mg daily. We recommend 150 to 600 mg magnesium citrate daily. Patients with high blood pressure may, under a doctor's direction, take up to 750 mg daily.

Manganese

If it worked on the stock exchange, manganese would be a runner—not as impressive as a trader, but just as necessary for the inner workings of the economy.

Manganese does not come with a long list of achievements or responsibilities, but it is necessary as a component of numerous enzymes for the metabolism of protein, fat, and carbohydrates. Most important for us is that this mineral enhances energy metabolism.

As a component of other substances, manganese aids the body in numerous functions. It protects cells because it is a component of superoxide dismutase (SOD), an important antioxidant that helps fight free radicals capable of causing cellular damage. It aids in fertility because it is needed for sperm motility. As a part of glucosamine, a substance that supports our joints, manganese helps to prevent and treat bone and joint problems.

Moreover, although research has not yet verified a correlation, numerous other ailments seem to appear routinely in people who have low amounts of manganese in their bodies. These include asthma, diabetes, and heart disease. It is document-ed and proven that a deficiency of manganese causes poor growth, impaired glu-cose tolerance (hence the diabetes suspicion), nervous system disorders, abnormal reproduction, protein-calorie malnutrition, and a weakened immune system.

Manganese occurs naturally in fruits, vegetables, legumes, oatmeal or bran, nuts, coffee, tea, and rice.

Dosage: The RDA for adults is 2-5 mg per day, but 35 mg can be ingested with-out toxicity. Only about 40 percent is absorbed, but you can up the absorption rate by consuming zinc and vitamin C.

Manganese should be taken in relation to zinc and copper; these minerals affect each other's absorption. Take two to five times the amount of zinc as manganese.

Muira Puama

It's a big mystery how his Brazilian shrub, also called "potency wood," actually succeeds in increasing sexual desire and erection. But a large number of men report a significant improvement in their sex drive and ability to get an erection after taking the extract for at least two weeks.

Reports state that the herb seems to affect men in psychological as well as phys-ical ways. It has long been used in South America as an aphrodisiac and nerve stimulant. There are reports that the herb has a positive effect on cognition and a recent study published in *Pharmacology, Biochemistry, and Behavior* found that it may have some use as a treatment for fighting cognitive decline.

In a study conducted by Dr. Jacque Waynberg, an expert on human sexual behavior at the Institute of Sexology in Paris, 100 men were given muira puama. Frequency of intercourse increased for 63 percent of these men, two-thirds said they were less fatigued overall, and 9 out of 10 said they felt less tired after sex.

And in a study presented at the First International Congress on Ethnopharmacology, 262 men with erectile problems were given 1 – 1.5 mg muira puama daily. Within 2 weeks, six out of ten reported improvements in their ability to achieve an erection.

Dosage: 1 to 1.5 grams daily.

For some reason, either genetics or environmental reasons (or both), we are hard-wired to respond to certain smells. Four of the top smells that increase blood flow to the penis are (1) lavender (2) licorice (3) chocolate and (4) pumpkin pie.

Nettles (Urtica Dioica)

The nettle fruit (what we commonly think of as the nettle itself), nettle leaf or herb, and nettle root are all considered functional herbs, but for our purposes the nettle root is most impressive.

The nettle root, or stinging nettle root, has been proved to effectively relieve symptoms of BPH stages 1 and 2. The root does not, in fact, reduce the size of the prostate, but it does reduce the congestion and difficulties of urination. There is speculation that the root has pharmacological components and that it somehow interferes with testosterone metabolism. An early study published in a 1983 issue of *Fortschr Med* concluded that nettles inhibit the binding of dihydrotesterone (the bad testosterone for BPH) with the receptors in the prostate—a bond which is thought to be the primary cause of BPH.

Based on current research, some European countries (including Germany, where much of the current research has been conducted) have formed what will hopefully become a bandwagon, approving the drug for treatment of prostatic diseases.

The nettle fruit and leaf are also considered by many herbalists to strengthen and support systems of the entire body. They are used as therapy for inflammatory diseases of the urinary tract and the prevention and treatment of kidney gravel. They are reported to be effective treatments for the symptoms of rheumatism, arthritis, eczema, hemorrhages of many kinds, diseases of the colon, and diarrhea.

Folk remedies using nettle fruit include crushed fruits applied externally for skin complaints and rheumatism. Cold-pressed oil attained from the fruit is given internally as a tonic to increase activity of the liver. The fruit is also used to treat diarrhea and biliary complaints.

Another folk remedy calls for nettle herb taken as a tea or juice internally to serve as a blood-forming agent, as a diuretic in arthritis and rheumatism of the joints and muscles. Nettle root has also been used as a diuretic, as an astringent and gargle.

One Warsaw School of Medicine (Poland) study found that nettle root combined with pygeum africanum bark extract significantly reduced urine flow, residual urine, and nycturia in patients with BPH. One

> **O**ne study suggests that combining stinging nettle with pygeum africanum may be effective in reducing the symptoms of benign prostate enlargements.

group was given 300 mg of nettle root extract and 25 mg pygeum africanum bark extract (the standard dosage of the preparation) while one group was given half the dosage. Both groups showed equal improvement, leading to the conclusion that a half dosage is as effective and safe as a full dosage.

Nettle dosages:

Stinging nettle herb and leaf: 8-12 g daily.

Stinging nettle root: 4-6 g daily.

Infusion: pour 1 cup of boiling water onto 3 teaspoons of the dried herb, infuse for 10-15 minutes, drink 3 times daily.*

Tincture: 1-4 ml of the tincture 3 times daily.

Side effects (occasional): upset stomach.

> **✱NOTE:** Personally, I prefer to take supplements as caplets rather than infusions or teas. Otherwise, I'd be running to the bathroom constantly!

Niacin (Nitotinic Acid, Vitamin B$_3$)

Energy! Energy! Energy! Niacin is necessary for the production of energy from glucose, and glucose is our primary source of energy. That makes niacin pretty important if we want to take a run, make love to our wife, get up in the morning, or even stay alive!

Niacin is a vasodilator, meaning it can help widen dilation of blood vessels, causing them to increase in size. That means that it helps with all circulation-related ailments of age, including senility (with is related to a lack of blood flow to the brain), circulatory ailments of the limbs, and circulation-related sexual problems, among others.

By promoting blood flow to the penis niacin may be able to help a man achieve and maintain erections. Also important for us guys, adequate levels of niacin are essential for the production of testosterone.

Niacin is important for those of us with weight or dietary concerns. It converts sugar and fat to energy, so it's an important vitamin for maintaining your ideal weight. Niaicin helps lower triglycerides (which are a kind of fat) and lipoprotein (which is a product of bad cholesterol that increases your risk of heart disease).

As you've no doubt heard, it is no longer enough to simply lower our cholesterol—now we have to know <u>which</u> kind is "good" and which is "bad." The bad cholesterol, LDL, can clog your arteries and give you a heart attack. The good kind is HDL cholesterol, which helps cleanse your system of the <u>bad</u> LDL. In one study niacin dropped LDL cholesterol levels by 17% and triglyceride levels by 18%, while raising HDL levels 16%.

Because of all of the above actions of niacin, it is considered to be a drug for effectively fighting and preventing heart disease. It is not widely prescribed, because in large dosages (and without the other B's) it causes various side effects, such as itching. But at the proper dosage, it can be a highly healthful vitamin largely without side effects.

Niacin is a coenzyme necessary for several cellular processes involving carbohydrate, fat, and protein metabolism; growth; digestion; and hormone synthesis. Derivative forms: niacinamide or nicotinamide.

Deficiency of niacin is called pellagra, which means "rough skin" in Italian. In the late 1930s, U.S. food manufacturers began to enrich bread with niacin to prevent pellagra. In addition to dermatitis and skin lesions that give pellagra its name, other symptoms can include depression, diarrhea, malfunctioning of the nervous system, and gastrointestinal upset. Niacin may play a role in treating atrial fibrillation (or other regular heartbeat symptoms), schizophrenia, and other mental illness.

CAUTION!

Be sure to consult your doctor before taking niacin if you suffer from any of the following conditions: diabetes, low blood pressure, liver disease, gout, ulcers, bleeding problems or glaucoma.

Time-released niacin was developed to counteract the skin-flushing side effect this B vitamin can cause. However studies have shown this form of the vitamin can be damaging to the liver and it's best to avoid it.

Niacin has been used, in large doses (500 to 1,000 mg or more daily) to lower levels of low-density (LDL) cholesterol, the "bad" cholesterol, as well as lower triglyceride levels. At the same time, it can raise the level of high-density lipoprotein (HDL), the "good" cholesterol. But these doses, which far exceed the RDA, can cause unpleasant and potentially dangerous side effects including skin rash, flushing, heartburn, nausea, elevated blood sugar, and in severe cases, liver damage.

Coffee contains niacin, and drinking coffee probably has prevented niacin deficiency in people with poor diets. Other foods that are good sources of niacin (or of tryptophan, an amino acid that can be converted to niacin in the body) include liver, kidney, poultry, beans, peas, tuna, halibut, fruits, grains, cereals, yeast, green leafy vegetables, cheese, milk, beef, carrots, broccoli, corn flour, potatoes, tomatoes, and eggs. Once consumed, niacin is rapidly absorbed in the stomach and intestine.

If you are diabetic, please do not take niacin unless your doctor OK's it. Yes, niacin can protect your arteries, but be aware that it <u>may</u> have the potential to also raise your blood sugar (the jury is still out on this one).

As suggested elsewhere in this book, it's best to take all your B vitamins together, especially if you want to reduce side effects. They were created in nature together, and your body wants them together.

Taking niacin supplements will probably make you flush, but that harmless reaction will lessen as you maintain use over time. Taking the supplement with food or an aspirin may help to reduce this effect.

The RDA for adults is 1 to 19 mcg "niacin equivalents," an equivalency based on preformed niacin. Each niacin equivalent is equal to one mg of preformed niacin.

Or take 100 mg of B_3 (in conjunction with the other B's). Generally, 500-1000 mg is used as a therapeutic dosage, but I personally forbid you from taking that much unless you are under the care of a doctor, who tells you that you may do so.

When taken with vitamin C, niacin reduces the risk of high lipoprotein levels. There is some preliminary evidence that taking chromium may make niacin effective at very low doses.

Nutmeg

Since Western societies generally use nutmeg solely for its pleasing scent and taste, we need to turn to other cultures to learn about the medicinal properties of this delicious herb.

Men in Yemen, for example, consume nutmeg to boost their sexual vigor and drive. The Hindu Pharmacopoeia recommends nutmeg as a treatment for fever, asthma, and heart disease. The Arabs used nutmeg over 1,200 years ago to treat digestive disorders, kidney disease, and lymphatic ailments. It is known to induce a mild sense of euphoria, which may explain nutmeg's reported ability to heighten sexual pleasure.

Nutmeg is a spice made from the seed of the nutmeg tree, a tropical evergreen that can grow to heights of 65 feet. The trees have bell-shaped flowers and bear a fleshy, lemon-yellow fruit. Inside the fruit, surrounded by a lacy membrane, is a hard, egg-shaped seed—grayish brown and about an inch long. The spice, made by grinding the seeds, has a pleasant fragrance and sweet, warm taste. It's a great ingredient in cooking and baking, used in squash, turnips, spinach, puddings, confections, baked goods, and cream-based dishes. Sniff a sachet and you'll likely smell nutmeg in the mix.

Nutmeg was one of the spices Christopher Columbus was searching for when he set sail from Spain to find the East Indies. Nutmeg was one of the most sought-after commodities in 17th century Europe, valued above gold for its powerful medicinal properties.

Warning: Myristicin, a toxic, crystalline, safrole derivative found in nutmeg, can cause vomiting, nausea, dry mouth, hallucinations, and convulsions if taken in large doses.

CAUTION!

If you are suffering from BPH you may want to avoid using nutmeg. Nutmeg may inhibit prostaglandin synthesis, which could cause your symptoms to worsen.

Octacosanol

Octacosanol is touted as a brain drug and energy booster (ginkgo, step aside!). It has been used to combat comas, brain disorders, fatigue, and to aid people with multiple sclerosis by increasing their energy. In addition it has been shown to significantly lower total cholesterol levels as well as low-density lipoprotein (LDL or "bad") cholesterol levels.

Although octacosanol has been studied no one knows quite why or how it works. But it sounds to me like it's worth learning about. An early 1972 study showed that wheat germ oil, of which octacosanol is a component, has proven to increase endurance and oxygen intake at high altitudes. Joined with other components (tri-acontanol, tetracosanol, and hexacosanol) of wheat germ oil, octacosanol displays the same effects as it does alone (and only in combination has it been studied as a booster of endurance and oxygen consumption).

Octacosnol's ability to lower cholesterol levels has been documented in randomized double blind studies. In a study published in the journal *International Journal of Tissue Reactions* octacosanol outperformed a prescription cholesterol-

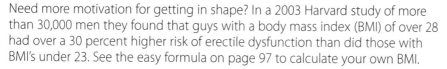

STUDY RESULTS

Need more motivation for getting in shape? In a 2003 Harvard study of more than 30,000 men they found that guys with a body mass index (BMI) of over 28 had over a 30 percent higher risk of erectile dysfunction than did those with BMI's under 23. See the easy formula on page 97 to calculate your own BMI.

Ann Intern Med. 2003 Aug 5;139(3):161-8.

Sexual function in men older than 50 years of age: results from the health professionals follow-up study.

Bacon CG, Mittleman MA, Kawachi I, Giovannucci E, Glasser DB, Rimm EB.

Department of Nutrition, Harvard School of Public Health, Brigham and Woman's Hospital, 665 Huntington Avenue, Boston, Massachusetts 02115, USA.

BACKGROUND: Although many studies have provided data on erectile dysfunction in specific settings, few studies have been large enough to precisely examine age-specific prevalence and correlates. OBJECTIVE: To describe the association between age and several aspects of sexual functioning in men older than 50 years of age. DESIGN: Cross-sectional analysis of data from a prospective cohort study. SETTING: U.S. health professionals. PARTICIPANTS: 31 742 men, age 53 to 90 years. MEASUREMENTS: Questionnaires mailed in 2000 asked about sexual function, physical activity, body weight, smoking, marital status, medical conditions, and medications. Previous biennial questionnaires since 1986 asked about date of birth, alcohol intake, and other health information. RESULTS: When men with prostate cancer were excluded, the age-standardized prevalence of erectile dysfunction in the previous 3 months was 33%. Many aspects of sexual function (including overall function, desire, orgasm, and overall ability) decreased sharply by decade after 50 years of age. Physical activity was associated with lower risk for erectile dysfunction (multivariable relative risk, 0.7 [95% CI, 0.6 to 0.7] for >32.6 metabolic equivalent hours of exercise per week vs. 0 to 2.7 metabolic equivalent hours of exercise per week), and obesity was associated with higher risk (relative risk, 1.3 [CI, 1.2 to 1.4] for body mass index >28.7 kg/m2 vs. <23.2 kg/m2). Smoking, alcohol consumption, and television viewing time were also associated with increased prevalence of erectile dysfunction. Men who had no chronic medical conditions and engaged in healthy behaviors had the lowest prevalence. CONCLUSIONS: Several modifiable health behaviors were associated with maintenance of good erectile function, even after comorbid conditions were considered. Lifestyle factors most strongly associated with erectile dysfunction were physical activity and leanness.

PMID: 12899583
[PubMed - indexed for MEDLINE]

lowering drug, dropping total cholesterol levels 15.8% compared to the prescription drugs 7.5% drop. In addition octacosanal dropped LDL cholesterol levels by 21% compared to 7.5% by the prescription medication!

Dosage: You can use a natural extract of wheat germ oil instead of octacosanol. Studies have used from 40-80 mg per day, but 15-20 mg per day should suffice.

Pantothenic Acid (Vitamin B₅)

From the sound of it (or should I say the <u>action</u> of it), I really like pantothenic acid. Discovered in 1940, this vitamin does lots of nice things that we need for good healthy activity, including sexual activity.

Also known as B_5, pantothenic acid, is an anti-oxidant for the adrenal system, and supports the production of steroids. In plain English, that means that it helps keep your hormone system in good health, supporting your body's sexual and metabolic functions, just to name two good ones. B_5 is involved in energy metabolism of carbohydrates, proteins, and lipids.

The adrenals also produce adrenaline and hormones that act as anti-inflammatories. For that reason, B_5 is considered to have important roles in disease-fighting and disease preventing, and may even help to calm anything you've got that's inflamed.

Vitamin B_5 is a key component of coenzyme A, which helps remove toxic substances from the body. Coenzyme A also converts carbohydrates, fats, and protein into energy.

Pantothenic acid supports normal functioning of the gastrointestinal tract and production of bile, vitamin D, red blood cells, and antibodies. It is known to improve glucose tolerance, increase cancer immunity, and fight fatigue. Some alternative medicine researchers believe pantothenic acid may even help get rid of gray hair.

By helping you produce acetylcholine, a neurotransmitter, pantothenic acid may help combat depression. Studies suggest that it may also be able to help lower cholesterol, and to reduce the levels of triglycerides and low-density lipoprotein (or LDL, the "bad" cholesterol), two dangerous fats in our blood. It simultaneously appears to raise high-density lipoprotein (or HDL, the "good" cholesterol). Thus it is used to prevent and to fight heart disease. It is also great for people who are recovering from heart surgery.

Pantothenic acid has been used for various skin ailments, and may help treat obesity (because it bolsters the creation of coenzyme A in your body, which decreases appetite, and which is naturally depleted in weight loss).

When taken with the other B vitamins, pantothenic acid's beneficial effects are increased, and the possible side effects of each B vitamin are reduced or eliminated. The B vitamins occur together naturally in the body, so taking them together as supplements replicates the natural environment more accurately.

Together with vitamins B_1, B_2, and B_3, pantothenic acid helps make ATP, the substance that gives your body its energy. With vitamin A, pantothenic acid is used for various skin ailments. With vitamin E, it is used to fight cholesterol build up.

Foods that are good sources of pantothenic acid include poultry, soybeans, yogurt, liver, kidney, brewer's yeast, blue cheese, sweet potatoes, salmon, vegetables, eggs, grain, seafood, beans, beef, brown rice, lobster, sunflower seeds, mushrooms, avocados, cauliflower, green peas, nuts, dates, and meat.

B_5 is soluble in water and cannot be stored in the body. That means you need a constant supply from food or supplements, or both.

Dosage: It is recommended that adults get from 10 mg of pantothenic acid daily. For supplementation, I recommend 100-200 mg per day. Take up to 500 mg per day to treat specific ailments only after checking with your doctor first.

Side Effects: Large doses of this supplement can occasionally cause diarrhea. Reduce your dosage if you experience this problem and be sure to tell your doctor about any side effects you have.

Your body mass index, or BMI, is a measurement of your weight in relation to your height. To calculate your own BMI divide your weight in pounds by your height in inches squared and then multiply by 703.

For example if you are 5 foot 7 (67 inches) and weigh 220 pounds you would calculate your BMI like this: 220 divided by 4489 (67" x 67") multiplied by 703 = 34.45 BMI.

Pygeum Africanum

In traditional African medicine a tea is made from the powder of the African evergreen tree called Pygeum Africanum to relieve urinary discomforts in men. Like saw palmetto, pygeum africanum is a pretty well known herb. It is often used

STUDY RESULTS

A systematic review of existing studies on pygeum africanum, published in the online journal *Cochrane Database of Systematic Reviews*, found that pygeum consistently and significantly outperformed placebos in relieving the symptoms of BPH. Men using the supplement were more than twice as likely to report an improvement in overall symptoms. Nighttime urination was reduced by 19%, residual urine volume by 24% and peak urine flow was increased by 23%.

Cochrane Database Syst Rev. 2002;(1):CD001044.

Pygeum africanum for benign prostatic hyperplasia.

Wilt T, Ishani A, Mac Donald R, Rutks I, Stark G.

General Internal Medicine (111-0), Minneapolis VA/VISN 13 Center for Chronic Disease Outcomes Research, One Veterans Drive, Minneapolis, Minnesota 55417, USA.

BACKGROUND: Benign prostatic hyperplasia (BPH), nonmalignant enlargement of the prostate, can lead to obstructive and irritative lower urinary tract symptoms (LUTS). The pharmacologic use of plants and herbs (phytotherapy) for the treatment of LUTS associated with BPH has been growing steadily. The extract of the African prune tree, Pygeum africanum, is one of the several phytotherapeutic agents available for the treatment of BPH.

OBJECTIVES: To investigate the evidence whether extracts of Pygeum africanum (1) are more effective than placebo in the treatment of Benign Prostatic Hyperplasia (BPH), (2) are as effective as standard pharmacologic BPH treatments, and (3) have less side effects compared to standard BPH drugs.

SEARCH STRATEGY: Trials were searched in computerized general and specialized databases (MEDLINE (1966-2000), EMBASE, Cochrane Library, Phytodok), by checking bibliographies, and by contacting relevant manufacturers and researchers.

SELECTION CRITERIA: Trials were eligible if they (1) were randomized (2) included men with BPH (3) compared preparations of Pygeum africanum (alone or in combination) with placebo or other BPH medications (4) included clinical outcomes such as urologic symptom scales, symptoms, or urodynamic measurements. Eligibility was assessed by at least two independent observers.

DATA COLLECTION AND ANALYSIS: Information on patients, interventions, and outcomes were extracted by at least two independent reviewers using a standard form. The main outcome measure for comparing the effectiveness of Pygeum africanum with placebo and standard BPH medications was the change in urologic symptoms scale scores. Secondary outcomes included change in urologic symptoms including nocturia and urodynamic measures (peak and mean urine flow, prostate size). The main outcome measure for adverse effects was the number of men reporting adverse effects.

MAIN RESULTS: A total of 18 randomized controlled trials involving 1562 men met inclusion criteria and were analyzed. Only one of the studies reported a method of treatment allocation concealment, though 17 were double-blinded. There were no studies comparing Pygeum africanum to standard pharmacologic interventions such as alpha-adrenergic blockers or 5-alpha reductase inhibitors. The mean study duration was 64 days (range, 30-122 days). Many studies did not report results in a method that permitted meta-analysis. Compared to men receiving placebo, Pygeum africanum provided a moderately large improvement in the combined outcome of urologic symptoms and flow measures as assessed by an effect size defined by the difference of the mean change for each outcome divided by the pooled standard deviation for each outcome (-0.8 SD [95% confidence interval (CI), -1.4, -0.3 (n=6 studies)]). Men using Pygeum africanum were more than twice as likely to report an improvement in overall symptoms (RR=2.1, 95% CI = 1.4, 3.1). Nocturia was reduced by 19%, residual urine volume by 24% and peak urine flow was increased by 23%. Adverse effects due to Pygeum Africanum were mild and comparable to placebo. The overall dropout rate was 12% and was similar between Pygeum Africanum (13%), placebo (11%) and other controls (8%).

REVIEWER'S CONCLUSIONS: A standardized preparation of Pygeum africanum may be a useful treatment option for men with lower urinary symptoms consistent with benign prostatic hyperplasia. However, the reviewed studies were small in size, were of short duration, used varied doses and preparations and rarely reported outcomes using standardized validated measures of efficacy. Additional placebo-controlled trials are needed as well as studies that compare Pygeum africanum to active controls that have been convincingly demonstrated to have beneficial effects on lower urinary tract symptoms related to BPH. These trials should be of sufficient size and duration to detect important differences in clinically relevant endpoints and use standardized urologic symptom scale scores.

PMID: 11869585
[PubMed - indexed for MEDLINE]

to relieve symptoms of benign prostatic hyperplasia (BPH) a swelling of the prostate bland that can lead to urinary complaints. Many men with BPH report that after taking the herb their symptoms tend to lessen or even disappear, including all urinary disorders associated with BPH. Actually, in a few different studies, patients even reported that their sexual performance was increased after taking the herb for over a month, too. This may simply be because they were feeling better in general after their urinary complaints were relieved, but what matters is that it worked for them.

All studies on pygeum have been performed using an extract of the bark. Medical folks call it the "standardized extract" because it combines the active ingredients in the amounts proven to be most effective. While additional randomized placebo controlled studies are needed to prove once and for all the effectiveness of this herb there is plenty of word of mouth support for its use.

Dosage: 5 to 100 mg of the extract can be taken twice daily.

Psoralea Seed (Psoralen)

You can call this "fruit of the scurfy pea" if you have trouble pronouncing the real name (try spelling it!). Information on it is surprisingly scarce, taking into account the possible benefits. Considering some of the positive anecdotal reports out there I think it's worth including here. This seed has been used primarily in Traditional Chinese Medicine (TCM) to treat impotence, premature ejaculation, spermatorrhea (involuntary discharge of semen without orgasm), frequent urination, and urinary incontinence. So for many older men, it's a good one to grow on your windowsill.

The seed has also used in TCM to aid in combating diarrhea and abdominal pain and for increasing blood flow (hence the affect on impotence), as an antibiotic, and for treating male pattern baldness.

Known in the United States (particularly with the Appalachians) as a good luck charm, this plant is said to ward off snakes and treat rheumatism. Psoralea has been used in combination with cuscutae and fructus alpiniae oxyphyllae to treat urinary frequency, and with juglandis regiae for premature ejaculation.

Dosage: 3 – 9 g daily (extract of seed). As a tea, two or three roots are used per quart of water and boiled for 30 minutes.

Pumpkin Seed

Did you realize that eating those roasted pumpkin seeds at Halloween could be indirectly helping your sex life? Pumpkin seeds, especially in combination with some other herbs, are thought to be an effective prostate helper. Now that is something to make any Jack O' Lantern smile!

If you check the ingredients list on a number of natural urological or prostate remedies you will probably find that pumpkin seed is often one of the ingredients listed. This is because of its effects on sex-hormone binding globulin (that's the substance whose malfunction is thought to lead to prostate problems in the first place).

DID YOU KNOW ?

Contrary to popular belief the more often people masturbate the more often they have sex. It's theorized that masturbating raises testosterone and dopamine levels putting you in the mood more often.

Specifically, it is believed to help with urination problems associated with BPH stages one and two. While there is no evidence that it will actually reduce the size of the prostate, there is plenty of empirical evidence that the zinc and amino acid packed pumpkin seed has an ability to improve the symptoms of BPH. Hey, sounds good to me for a safe, natural, not to mention tasty remedy.

Dosage: 10-20 g of seed daily.

Pycnogenol (Grape Seed Extract)

Chances are you have read or heard at least something about pycnogenol, which can be extracted from pine bark, grape seed, and other fruits. It is known by many names including OPC (oligomeric procyanidins), proanthocyanidolic oligomers, and grape seed extract.

Pycnogenol is a powerful antioxidant weighing in at 50 times stronger than vitamin E, and 20 times stronger than vitamin C. Wow, that's some powerful stuff!

French and Japanese clinical studies have shown that pycnogenol may help the body resist damage and inflammation of the skin and blood vessels, partly by binding to and preventing the destruction of collagen. Studies suggest that pycnogenol may strengthen the circulatory system, including arteries and small vessels (and I don't need to remind you what part of your body depends on good blood flow for

STUDY RESULTS

If eating pumpkin seeds doesn't help your sex life, try baking a pumpkin pie. A study of 31 men ages 18 to 64, conducted by Dr. Alan Hirsh, neurologist and psychiatrist of the Smell & Taste Treatment and Research Foundation in Chicago, found that the smell of pumpkin pie and lavender together increased blood flow to the penis by 40 percent. No one has any idea why. Some theorize that possibly pleasant early memories may be associated with the scents.

Various Aromas Found to Enhance Male Sexual Response

Hirsch Alan, Gruss Jason
The Smell and Taste Treatment and Research Foundation, Chicago

Objective: Folk wisdom suggests that various aromas are sexually enticing, but no data exists demonstrating the actual effects of specific odors on arousal. Dr. Hirsch and colleague Dr. Jason Gruss initiated a study to investigate the impact of ambient olfactory stimuli upon sexual response in the human male.

Methods:

1) The team recruited volunteers literate in English through solicitation on classic rock radio broadcasts. Thirty-one men, aged 18 to 64 years, signed up.

2) All subjects underwent olfactory testing with the University of Pennsylvania Smell Identification Test (UPSIT), a 40-item, forced choice, scratch and sniff odor detection and identification test. They were queried on sexual preference, sexual practices and odor preferences.

3) Dr. Hirsch selected 24 different odorants for the study. In addition, six combinations of two of the most well-liked of these were also chosen.

4) The effects of the 30 odors on penile blood flow were assessed by comparing a subject's brachial penile index while wearing an odorized mask to his average index while wearing an unodorized mask. This was done for each subject for each odor.

5) The men underwent assessment as follows: After being attached to a plethysmograph (which measures penile blood flow), three minutes were allowed for acclimation. Then a blank, nonodorized mask was applied for one minute while a baseline brachial penile index was recorded.

6) After the blank mask was removed, an odorized mask was applied. Thus, 30 odorized masks were randomly applied in double-blind fashion, with a three-minute hiatus between masks to prevent habituation of the odors. Each mask was worn for one minute while brachial penile index was recorded.

7) Finally, an additional blank mask was applied for one minute and brachial penile index once again recorded.

Results: Each of the 30 odors produced an increase in penile blood flow.

Increase in Penile Blood Flow Produced by Top 10 Odors in 31 Male Volunteers

Odor or odor combination	Average Increase
Lavender and pumpkin pie	40%
Doughnut & black licorice	31.5%
Pumpkin pie & doughnut	20%
Orange	19.5%
Lavender & doughnut	18%
Black licorice and cola	13%
Black licorice	13%
Doughnut & cola	12.5%
Lily of the valley	11%
Buttered popcorn	9%

However, not all increased arousal to the same degree. The combined odor of lavender and pumpkin pie had the greatest effect, increasing median penile blood flow by 40%. Next in effectiveness was the combination of black licorice and doughnut, which increased arousal by 31.5%. And so on, all the way down to cranberry, which only increased penile

blood flow by 2%. Depending on the man's age, they may have reacted differently than their counterparts to certain smells. For instance, older men tended to respond strongly to vanilla.

Conclusion: Dr. Hirsch's team theorized that pleasant odors, since they tend to positively increase other behaviors, would likely increase penile blood flow. Their data supported this hypothesis. However, a multitude of mechanisms could be at play. The odors could induce a Pavlovian conditioned response reminding partners of sexual partners or their favorite foods. Odors could have evoked nostalgic recall. Or the odors may simply be relaxing. The odors could also awaken the reticular activating system, making the men more alert to any sexual cues, thus increasing penile blood flow. The odors may also act neurophysiologically. A direct pathway connects the olfactory bulb to the septal nucleus, which in turn induces blood flow and erection. Other possible explanations exist, but the direct connection between odors and sexual response cannot be denied. Homologous studies on vaginal blood flow have also been carried out.

peak sexual health!). One French study showed a 25 percent increase in capillary strength in patients taking grape seed OPC. It has even been suggested that pycnogenol may have a protective effect on brain cells slowing memory loss.

Pycnogenol has also been used to fight atherosclerosis and arthritis because is thought to stimulate connective tissue. Positive effects include decreased heartbeat, improved sleep and mood, and even relief of tennis elbow.

Dosage: Grape seed extract is generally considered to be superior to pycnogenol that comes from pine bark because of its slightly higher concentration—98 percent for grape seed vs. 95 percent for pine—of OPC. The standard dosages for pycnogenol and grape seed extract are comparable, with both at 150 – 300 mg daily for most ailments.

Caution: Although circulatory problems may require more OPC, you should check with your doctor before exceeding 300 mg per day.

Pyridoxine (Vitamin B$_6$)

Like the rest of the B vitamins B$_6$ is vital to our health. It is crucial for the metabolism of amino acids and more than 60 enzymes in the body. The production of many hormones, and also the production of serotonin (that's the chemical in your brain that makes you feel happy) require B$_6$.

Pyridoxine is necessary for our brains to function properly because it is needed for the production of neurotransmitters, which are like the communicators in the brain. Neurotransmitters actually make it possible for information to travel from brain neuron to brain neuron.

Because so many functions rely on it, it's no wonder that pyridoxine has also proven to treat numerous ailments. It lowers a type of hemoglobin that's associated with diabetes damage, indicating that it may treat some of the damage from this disease. It also has been shown in some cases to stabilize blood sugar.

In addition, pyridoxine plays an important role in the prevention and treatment of heart disease by helping to clear clogged arteries and blood vessels, and by helping to reduce or eliminate homocysteine, an amino acid which has been shown to exist in high levels in people who have heart attacks or strokes.

B$_6$ also strengthens the immune system in general, which means of course that it aids our body in fighting off any ailment or disease. In fact, a lack of B$_6$ diminishes our levels of T cells, which are the body's gauge of immune function. (Think of these cells as soldier's defending your body from viruses and other invaders. The more soldiers on your side, the more likely your army is to win the battle.) B$_6$ has been shown to be effective in combating a number of ailments ranging from asthma to skin disorders from appendage pain to kidney stones.

B$_6$ needs riboflavin to convert into its functional coenzyme in the body. It is best when taken in combination with the other B vitamins. When combined with magnesium orthophosphate, it reduces the likelihood of formation of kidney stones. In combination with folic acid and B$_{12}$, it may help prevent heart disease.

Of the B vitamin family, niacin (B$_3$), pyridoxine (B$_6$) and vitamin B$_{12}$ have been associated with improvements in circulation, reduction of prolactin (which helps to slow BPH), and support of adequate sperm production. In one study, a Harvard School of Public Health research team found that increasing vitamin B$_6$ consumption by only 2 mg daily reduced heart disease risk by 17%.

B$_6$ occurs naturally in pork and organ meats, whole wheat, oatmeal, wheat germ (the refinement of grains that occurs in many commercial products removes the B$_6$), legumes, and some fruits. Be aware that organ meats, while rich in B$_6$, are high in cholesterol.

Dosage: While the RDA for B$_6$ is 1 to 2 mg per day, many sources consider this to be a very low dosage. Studies have been done using 50 mg as a standard daily dosage and up to 200 mg per day for treatment of specific ailments (but check with your doctor if you want to take higher dosages).

Warning: Toxicity has occurred from taking 2 to 6 grams per day consistently over an extended period of time. Symptoms include sensory loss and numbness of the hands and feet. Side effects of all B vitamins are significantly reduced or eliminated if the B-complex vitamins are taken together.

TIPS

So much focus is put on the act of penetration itself that this pressure alone can cause anxiety and performance issues. Why not take the pressure off the "act" by making a commitment with your partner to delay penetration as long as possible in your next lovemaking session? Instead concentrate on finding at least 10 hot spots on your partner's body that drive her wild. Slow everything down to a crawl and concentrate on her reactions to your kisses and touches for clues when you are getting it right.

Royal Jelly

Produced by glands in the heads of worker bees, royal jelly is the bee version of the first batch of postpartum mother's milk—it gives bee larvae a mega-dose of life-sustaining nutrients to ensure the new bee's survival. Larvae destined to be queens are given two and a half days' extra dosage (which doubtless accounts for the name we've given it), aiding the she-monarchs in attaining their size, stamina, longevity, and boundless fertility.

Although I can't promise that royal jelly will help you sire an entire kingdom, this dynamo is remarkable in that it contains every basic nutrient integral in supporting life—both bee and human. It is a powerhouse of B vitamins, and of minerals such as calcium, iron, potassium, and silicon. It contains enzyme precursors, sex hormones, and many essential amino acids.

A natural antibiotic, royal jelly stimulates the immune system and promotes deep cellular health and longevity. Humans can use it to help build and rejuvenate their systems because it is said to create or stimulate energy and mental alertness.

In addition, the jelly is a rich source of pantothenic acid, which has been shown to combat stress, fatigue, and insomnia. The nutrients it provides are also essential for proper digestion, healthy skin, and hair.

> ## CAUTION!
>
> If you are allergic to bees you of course should steer clear of any bee related products. But even if you have never been diagnosed with an allergy to bees or bee pollen since bee products can lead to allergic reactions in some people its best to begin with small amounts to determine if you have an adverse reaction to them. Be on the look out for an itchy throat, wheezing, headaches, or hives and stop using the product immediately if you notice any of these side effects.

For those of us with a history of prostate difficulties, royal jelly may help directly with related hormone problems. It has been shown to be effective in the treatment of some prostate-related gland and hormone imbalances.

The Chinese, recognizing royal jelly's ability to increase a person's overall vitality, included it in their Precious Mirror of Health formula created in the 13th century.

Dosage: As little as one drop of pure, extracted royal jelly provides a full day's adequate supply. It is most effective when taken in its fresh or "alive" state; but it is also available and effective when taken in capsules in freeze dried form.

Sarsaparilla (Smilax Officinalis)

In Western movies, screenwriters often had the good guy walk into the bar and order sarsaparilla. This was meant to symbolize purity, since sarsaparilla in carbonated water is a non-alcoholic root beer-like soda. What those Hollywood types probably didn't realize was that sarsaparilla may have been giving those good guys a jump start to their potency as well.

In the past sarsaparilla has mostly been pigeon-holed as an aid for skin diseases, especially psoriasis. While it has been shown to have positive effects for a number of skin related conditions for our purposes the best benefits of the root of this climbing vine involve much more than just the skin. This herb excites me particularly because it has constituents that aid in the testosterone activity in the body. We like substances that help our testosterone activity!

In human studies, sarsaparilla has been shown to be a diuretic. (This may be an important point for any BPH sufferers out there). It can also help reduce itching, particularly of the anal region. In studies with animals it has been shown to protect the liver by boosting the immune system, and to be an anti-inflammatory (meaning it will potentially calm anything that's irritated or swollen).

It has also been listed in various medical and herbal sources for treatment of syphilis, herpes, and numerous skin disorders and diseases.

For psoriasis, it combines well with burdock, yellow dock and cleavers.

Dosage: dried root: 1-4 g daily. Liquid extract: (1:1 in 20% alcohol, 10% glycerol) 8-15ml daily.

Saw Palmetto (Serenoa Repens)

The word "saw" in the name of this short, shrubby palm refers to the thin, jagged-edged leaves resembling tiny saws. But the medicinal property is actually in the berry, not the leaves.

Numerous European clinical studies indicate that an extract of the fatty materials in the saw palmetto berry may be one of our best herbal treatments of BPH. The common theory is that BPH involves the accumulation of a certain sort of testosterone within the prostate, which causes prostate cells to multiply excessively. This gathering of the hormone where it doesn't belong causes the symptoms that many men have to suffer: an enlarged prostate gland, various urination difficulties, and sexual function disorders.

The appropriate extract (see below) of serenoa appears to inhibit the unwanted hormone components from binding with corresponding components (androgen receptors) in the prostate gland. In other words, it seems to aid in processes that may prevent the accumulation of the bad testosterone (dihydrotestosterone).

There are a whole bunch of studies showing the benefits of saw palmetto against BPH, suggesting that it is effective in up to 90 percent of patients, usually in 4 to 6 weeks. A study published in the journal *Rozhl Chir* showed that serenoa extract counteracted urination disorders and reduced prostate size (urinary flow, residuals, and prostate volume) associated with BPH. Results based on patients' recordings of symptoms and quantitative measurements suggest that serenoa extract is an effective treatment of various aspects of BPH.

And in a study published in the *British Journal of Clinical Pharmacology*, 55 men with an enlarged prostate who took 320 mg saw palmetto daily for a month had their urine flow improve five times better than a control group taking a placebo.

Saw palmetto has also traditionally been used to strengthen the male reproductive system in general. It is used for anything for which a boost in the male sex hormones is required. It is used as a diuretic (which means it will make you pee more easily), to reduce disease-causing microorganisms in the urinary tract, as an aid to the endocrine system (that's your hormones) specifically the sex-related hormones, and to prevent testicle disorders.

Saw palmetto has long been recognized as an effective sexual stimulant and aphrodisiac. To have great sex, both the man and women need a certain level of testosterone in the bloodstream (the man obviously needs more than the woman). Saw palmetto inhibits androgen and estrogen receptor activity, and can aid both sexes in achieving an optimal balance of sex hormones.

Saw palmetto is native to the Americas, and has been used as a tonic as long ago as the earliest Mayan civilizations. It has been used in western medicine since the mid-1800s, when articles were published supporting its effectiveness on body weight, general health, appetite stimulation, and reproductive health. Saw palmetto works well with damiana and kola for support of the reproductive system.

Dosage: 1-2 g saw palmetto berry; dried fruit: 0.5-1.0 g. Or put fi-1 teaspoons of berries in 1 cup of water, bring to boil, simmer gently for 5 minutes, and drink 3 times daily. Liquid extract: 0.6-1.5 ml daily. Tincture: 1-2 ml, 3 times daily. Note: The standard extract of saw palmetto used to treat BPH contains 85-95% fatty acids and may be effective at 160 mg twice daily.

Side effects: upset stomach (rare)

Schizandra Seed

The effects of Schizandra seed on the body are a lot like a milder form of ginseng. So why consider it? Well, if you're worried about particularly strong herbs (even those thought to be safe like ginseng), schizandra may be good for you. It has positive effects, but they may not be as pronounced as those you might get with ginseng. Like ginseng, schizandra seed is known as an adaptogen, which means it helps your body adapt—it regulates your body's functions to make them work well under stressors of different kinds. It also increases endurance and reduces gastric acidity.

If you have various sperm-related problems, it may help you, too. It's used for nocturnal emission (which has nothing to do with driving at night; it means letting loose sperm as you snooze), and prevents non-orgasmic release of sperm during the day too. In some cases it has been reported to help prevent excessive urination.

Widely used in China, it is thought to calm the spirit and is used for forgetfulness and insomnia. The seed has been recommended in combination with fructus psoraleae corylifoliae for chronic dysentery-like disorders and diarrhea caused by kidney disorders.

There is no standard documented dosage. Begin with a tiny amount, and gradually increase, noting how you feel. Do not exceed 10 g (.35 ounces) per 1 kg (2.21 pounds) of body weight daily; doses at 10 –15 kg per kg of body weight can cause toxicity.

Selenium

Minerals are interesting to me. I always get this picture in my head of shiny metals, or dirt-encrusted ore, when I think of a mineral. I guess it attests to our contemporary separation from the earth (or maybe I should speak for myself) that we think of our bodily matter as different from the matter of the land.

Any way you look at it, selenium is one impressive mineral. It's one of our most powerful antioxidants, which means it keeps our cells clean, protecting us from all sorts of diseases and ailments. Selenium is found primarily in the liver, kidneys, and heart, and acts as a protector of these important organs.

In numerous international studies, selenium has been shown to counteract heart disease. Studies show that people with low levels of selenium have a 70 percent greater risk of coronary heart disease than those with normal levels. Its antioxidant properties are responsible for this, but so is the fact that selenium limits the body's containment of cadmium, mercury, lead, and other toxic minerals that may harm tissues of the heart. It also protects the heart against low levels of oxygen.

Selenium can help combat many forms of cancer. A study published in the *Journal of the American Medical Association* found that 1,312 volunteers who took 200 mcg of selenium daily had their risk of contracting lung, prostate, and colorectal cancers cut in half.

Numerous national and international studies corroborate the conclusion of this study, as well as epidemiological evidence, which shows an increase in many kinds of cancer in areas where selenium levels in the soil (and therefore in foods eaten from the soil) are low. Selenium works with vitamin E as a cellular antioxidant; the mineral and vitamin depend on each other for many of their beneficial properties.

A landmark 10-year study, conducted by the University of Arizona, followed 1312 people living in areas of the USA that have low levels of selenium in the soil. The study, originally intended to look at the mineral's effect on skin cancer, yielded some surprising results. The researchers were shocked when they found that a daily selenium supplement could cut your overall risk of getting cancer by an incredible 50 percent. Men in the study, who were given 200 micrograms of selenium a day, had a 63 percent reduction in their risk of prostate cancer compared to those who received a placebo. The head researcher on the study, Dr. Larry Clark, speculated in a later interview that a particular protein found in the prostate is responsive to selenium and probably helps to protect the prostate against oxidative damage. Also significant was the fact that the selenium treated group had 46 percent fewer lung cancers, 58 percent fewer colorectal cancers, and half as many deaths from cancer.

Foods rich in selenium include brazil nuts, tuna, oysters, mackerel, wheat germ, sunflower seeds, turkey, shrimp, chicken breast, brown rice, and oatmeal.

Dosage: The recommended daily allowance (RDA) for men is 70 micrograms (mcg) daily, but studies have shown impressive results using 200 mcg daily.

Side effects: In normal dosages none have been reported. At excessive dosages of 500 mcg or more daily dry, peeling nails and skin; hair loss; nausea; diarrhea; fatigue; and bad breath.

Warning: at 125 times the RDA, selenium can cause toxicity, nervous system impairment, fatigue, nausea, and vomiting.

Thiamine (Vitamin B$_1$)

This important B vitamin helps convert carbohydrates into energy and enhances production of hydrochloric acid, the acid in your stomach that breaks down food. It is essential for maintaining the proper functioning of your nervous system, heart, muscles, brain, and coordination. It's easy to see how this translates to your sex life.

Deficiency of thiamine can contribute to eye weakness, loss of physical coordination, mental confusion, memory loss, irritability, fatigue, loss of appetite, constipation, shingles, anemia, moodiness, blood clots, heart muscle degeneration, and in severe cases beriberi, a potentially fatal disease of the central nervous system. Alcoholics are especially susceptible to thiamine deficiency.

A water-soluble nutrient, thiamine can't be stored in your body, so daily intake is required. Foods rich in thiamine include dried beans, eggs, brewer's yeast, whole grains, brown rice, seafood, artichokes, asparagus, watercress, cabbage, radishes, coconut, grapefruit, pineapple, almonds, filberts, peanuts, hazelnuts, bacon, ham, beef heart, lamb, liver, rye, and wheat germ.

Dosage: RDA 1.5 mg daily, though 50 to 500 mg daily is more typical for many Americans. Excess thiamine is excreted from the body.

Trigonella Seeds / Fenugreek

Well, fenugreek won't help you get it up, but it may treat other important health problems that threaten your well being as a whole, including diabetes—a disease causing impotency in many men.

Fenugreek has been shown to have the ability to reduce blood sugar in both diabetics and people without the disease. In Type I and Type II diabetes, it has been shown to reduce blood fats and blood sugars. This in turn lowers fasting glucose levels, improving glucose tolerance and insulin responses. Fenugreek also reduces serum cholesterol levels and the amount of urinary glucose secretion.

There is an indication, in tests with animals, that trigonella has steroidal effects. The seeds to do contain steroid saponins which have been shown to reduce blood cholesterol levels and to increase appetite (as steroids often do). Steroids help in the production of hormones, thereby supplying energy to our body's glands and organs so they can function effectively. So, this stuff may have a similar action to wild yam—it may bolster your hormone system, thereby also bolstering your sexual health.

Some Indian and Eastern cultures attribute aphrodisiac properties to the herb as well. Turkish men and women say that it increases their sexual potency.

Dosage: Standard daily dosage is 6 g. A tea can be taken several times a day. To prepare an infusion, leave 0.5 g of trigonella in cold water for three hours. Strain. A poultice (hot compress) can be made from powdered seeds and hot water (50 g per 1 liter of water) to treat skin inflammation or complaints.

For treatment of diabetes, 25 to 100 g per day of the ground seeds has been given. No health risks or side effects have been observed with the standard therapeutic dosage of 6 grams, but you should consult your doctor if you plan to take the large amount designated for diabetes.

Vitamin A

Vitamin A comes in two forms. The first is retinol, which is the "preformed" type, meaning it exists as a complete vitamin when you ingest it. Entering your body already complete, it allows your body to absorb 80 percent to 90 percent of the nutrient.

The second kind is carotene, which is a "provitamin." That means that carotene exists as an incomplete vitamin, but allows your body to convert it into a complete vitamin. Your body absorbs about 33 percent of this form.

Unabsorbed vitamins are stored primarily in the liver, kidneys, and fat tissue, and aren't harmful. But you might want to take in to account how much of what you ingest is actually being used. If you take in carotene, only 33 percent is working for you. That's why a standard RDA of "vitamin A" would be inaccurate—how much you actually use depends on what kind you ingest.

That said the majority of the vitamin A that we typically ingest comes from carotene, because it is in that form that it most often exists naturally. Your body will only store the unused parts of the vitamin for up to a year, so don't get visions in your head of your vital organs crammed with vitamin A—that won't happen.

Vitamin A is necessary for good vision, bone growth, and health of epithelial tissue, which is the cellular covering of internal and external organs, including passageways that link the inside to the outside of the body (so we're talking mouth, urinary canal, etc.). But most importantly for our purposes, vitamin A is necessary for energy regulation. Vitamin A metabolizes into retinoic acid, which aids in our body's production of heat and regulation of energy.

Newer research also suggests that vitamin A and carotene may help prevent heart disease and various forms of cancer, and bolster the beneficial effects of current cancer-fighting treatments.

Vitamin A and essential fatty acids (also found in pumpkin seeds) have also been recommended for optimum sexual health. They can usually be attained through the combination of a good diet and a high-quality multiple vitamin/mineral formula. Specific missing nutrients can then be added if there is an increased need for them, depending on your physiology and the contents of the multivitamin you choose.

Most vitamins work best in combination with each other. Vitamin A works well with other antioxidants (vitamin E, vitamin C, carotenoids) to fight cancer, prevent infections, and keep you in good health. It also often appears in medical studies in conjunction with selenium for treatment of many of the same ailments for which vitamin A is used alone.

Dosage: Vitamin A has to be ingested through the diet. Retinol (the complete kind, that you absorb a lot of) can be found in whole milk, cream, butter, eggs, and organ meats (like liver). But the majority of vitamin A found in typical American diets is obtained from carotene. This form of vitamin A can be detected because of its yellow/orange color—it is contained in carrots, sweet potatoes, squash, cantaloupe, and apricots. You can also find it in green vegetables, including spinach, collard greens, cabbage, broccoli, and other dark leafy greens.

The RDA of vitamin A is based on an equivalency measurement of retinol. A certain number of "retinol equivalents" means the amount of any vitamin A substance that will allow your body to use as much as one microgram of retinol. So the RDA is 800 mcg of retinol equivalents for women and 1000 mcg of retinol equivalents for men.

If you find this confusing (and I must admit I did at first) and you prefer the standard vitamin measurement, most adults should consume 5,000 International Units (IU) per day. For specific illnesses, you can take up to 100,000 IU per day, a dosage for which no side effects have been documented.

Cautions: Unlike most other vitamins, it is possible to ingest too much vitamin A from food alone—a condition that results in toxicity (called hypervitaminosis A). Signs of vitamin A toxicity include blurred vision, headaches, pains in the joints and bones, and poor appetite.

In rare cases, vitamin A supplements have caused liver failure, and in one documented case, death. (However, I must throw in here that this hasn't kept the FDA from approving vitamin A-derived drugs that deliver to the body quite hefty amounts of the vitamin, including the widely distributed patented commercial acne drug Accutane.)

Carotenemia is the condition that results from ingesting too much carotene. It can make your skin turn yellow, but it will go away within a few weeks if you reduce your intake.

Vitamin C (Ascorbic Acid)

As an antioxidant, vitamin C helps protect the body against free radical damage from any number of environmental sources in addition to the body's inherent metabolic byproducts. Our modern environment contributes to our free radical load when we are exposed to cigarette smoke, ionizing radiation, chemotherapy drugs, air pollution, pesticides, solvents, or formaldehyde.

How much? Each year, the U.S. produces more than 500 billion pounds of industrial wastes. That's more than one ton for every person. Dr. Ed Lemmo, a pioneering nutritional scientist, calls these substances "inadvertent contaminants"—pollutants that invade the air we breathe, the water we drink, the foods we eat, the very earth we live on. And in a study published in *Science News*, Dr. Arnold Schecter of New York State University concluded that every single person in the United States has detectable levels of toxic environmental solutions in their body tissues.

Sperm are extremely sensitive to free radicals because of their dependence on the integrity and fluidity of their cell membranes. Free radical damage can lead to impaired sperm motility, abnormal structure, less viability and finally the death of the sperm.

Vitamin C, beta-carotene, selenium, and vitamin E are all antioxidants that help protect against heart disease, cancer, sperm abnormalities, and infertility in men. They are also believed to slow the aging process and have long been associated with more satisfying sexual experiences. For purposes of optimal health, these nutrients can be elevated by changing your diet or taking supplements.

In addition to fighting free radicals on its own, vitamin C prevents other antioxidant vitamins, including A and E, from being oxidized, increasing their bioavailability and efficacy.

As we discussed in chapter 1, atherosclerosis and heart disease are major causes of impotence. In one study, patients with atherosclerosis were given 1,000 mg daily of vitamin C. They could soon walk farther without pain or becoming winded than a control group not receiving the vitamin. Another study, published in the journal *Circulation*, looked at carotid artery wall thickness in over 11,000 study participants and confirmed that vitamin C is indeed associated with a reduced risk of atherosclerosis. A study published in the journal *Epidemiology* demonstrated the for every 0.5 mg. per deciliter increase in blood levels of vitamin C there was an 11% drop in coronary heart disease as well as a reduction in strokes in a group of over 6,000 U.S. men and women. When the group was compared to individuals with low or marginal levels of C, there was a 27% reduction in heart disease and a 26% reduction in stroke in the group with the highest blood levels of vitamin C.

Stress, of course, can be a powerful inhibitor of male sexual performance. But C might be able to help in this department as well. A study from the University of Alabama, headed up by Samuel Campbell, suggests that taking vitamin C can reduce the level of stress hormones in the blood. When Dr. Campbell and his colleagues found that vitamin C not only reduced the stress hormones, but also reduced other typical indicators of stress such as weight loss, enlarged adrenal glands, and changes in the thymus and spleen in the test animals.

Vitamin C helps the body produce lymphocytes, which are the body's immune cells. It also helps transport phagocytes, protective cells that attack and destroy bacteria, viruses, cancer, and other foreign bodies.

Vitamin E

In all the hype about vitamin E—and there is certainly a lot of it out there—I bet you've never heard it called the man's vitamin. Me neither, but that's the way I'll think of it from now on, because it turns out that vitamin E enhances the ability of sperm to fertilize an egg in vitro, is the primary antioxidant for sperm membranes, and is a prominent component of the prostate gland. This on top of all the other more familiar benefits of this cleansing vitamin!

Because of its protection of red blood cells, vitamin E is a known heart disease fighter. In fact, it can help to keep arteries from clogging, lower bad cholesterol, raise good cholesterol, and lower triglycerides (a bad blood fat).

Numerous studies document vitamin E's ability to control "bad" (LDL) cholesterol. How does it work? vitamin E gets absorbed by the LDL particles, preventing them from sticking to blood vessel walls. This protects you against "hardening of the arteries" and the associated risk of heart attack. And of course, as you know, a healthy heart is a vital part of a healthy sex life: strong heart, strong arteries, strong erections.

In a University of Cambridge study, half of a population of 2,000 patients with confirmed heart disease, including a history of heart attack, were given 400 or 800 IU of vitamin E. The other 1,000 patients, in a control group, received a placebo. The group of patients taking vitamin E had an astounding 77 percent lower incidence of heart attack than those taking the placebo.

In a different study at the University of Mississippi, researchers fed monkeys a high-fat lard-cholesterol diet to block their arteries. Monkeys who got vitamin E in the study had 60 to 80 percent less artery clogging than those who did not. In addition, those monkeys who were given 108 IU of vitamin E daily after their

> **Y**our medical history can play an important part in your sexual functioning. If you have, or have had in the past, any of the following conditions it's important that your doctor and/or counselor is aware of it. All of them can contribute to a physical cause for impotence.
>
> 1. High blood pressure
> 2. Heart disease
> 3. Heart attack
> 4. Diabetes
> 5. Thyroid gland disease
> 6. Testicular disease
> 7. Multiple sclerosis
> 8. Parkinson's disease
> 9. Other neurological disease
> 10. Stroke
> 11. Kidney disease
> 12. Cancer

arteries clogged cleared their artery blockage by about 60 percent within 24 months.

As an overall health booster vitamin E is known to aid many of the body's processes, and to help prevent cancer, lung disease, arthritis, and blood disease. In its role as an antioxidant, it is a general immune system booster. Like many other immune system supporters, it has even been touted as an anti-aging vitamin, helping your entire body to maintain its vitality.

In a study of 29,000 Finnish men, the National Cancer Institute found that taking 50 IU (International Units) of vitamin E daily reduced their prostate cancer risk by one-third. And in a study at Columbia University the progression of Alzheimer's disease was significantly slowed in patients taking 2,000 IU daily of vitamin E for 2 years. And for you smokers out there several studies have drawn a connection between low vitamin E levels and prostate cancer risk in men.

Vitamin E occurs naturally in vegetable oils, whole grains, milk, eggs, meats, fish, and leafy vegetables. Normal cooking won't destroy it, but frying will (and we all know we really shouldn't be trying to pass off fried food as part of a healthy diet anyway). Commercial treatment of most of these foods, like hydrogenation of oil and enrichment or refinement of bread products, eliminates the vitamin (and most other healthy naturally occurring ingredients).

Dosage: RDA is 8-10 mg of "alpha-tocopherol equivalents" (that's the equivalent of 1 mg of naturally occurring vitamin E). As a supplement, 400-1200 IU per day is standard, and up to 3200 IU per day is safe.

Caution: More than 600 mg of alpha-tocopherol (an alcohol made from vitamin E) daily over an extended period of time may cause you to bleed excessively, impair your body's ability to heal wounds and may cause depression.

Yohimbe

"Beware! Danger! Tell your readers to consult their doctor!" says my conscience. I must admit that this stuff makes me a bit nervous.

Yohimbe can do wonderful things for sexual dysfunction, but we can reasonably apply the adage that the things that help you the most can hurt you the most too. The only FDA-approved drug for impotence before the times of Viagra, the alkaloid derived from yohimbe bark (called yohimbine) has been proven to improve sexual function by increasing blood flow to the penis.

Yohimbine is an alkaloid monoamine oxidase (MAO) inhibitor that blocks alpha-2 adrenergic receptors. This causes blood vessels to dilate, lowering blood pressure and increasing blood flow to erectile tissue.

Yohimbine also triggers and maintains neuroendocrine response in the hypothalmus to stimulate arousal psychogenically (meaning it makes you want to—which is nice, given the typical complaint that Viagra will technically get you up but won't really turn you on).

An article published in *The American Journal of Natural Medicine* states that yohimbine is successful in 34% to 43% of cases, and that it is effective in treating both the psycho-emotional and organic causes of impotence. In another study, four out of ten men who had been impotent for less than 2 years reported significant improvement in sexual performance after taking yohimbe for one month.

Researchers conducting double-blind, placebo-controlled studies report measurable improvements in libido and sexual performance in the men receiving the yohimbe vs. the placebo. Recent evidence suggests yohimbe may also aid in weight loss by suppressing the body's ability to store fat.

But yohimbe does unfortunately, like prescription impotence drugs, carry with it an impressive array of possible adverse side effects and health warnings. Most primary sources on yohimbe will suggest that people take it only under the guidance of a doctor. If you have heart, kidney, or liver problems, or nervous disorders like schizophrenia, don't take yohimbe. On the other hand, if you don't have any of these problems, you may want to try yohimbe with the help of a doctor or naturopath. Yohimbe tends to be really effective on the men for whom it works at all. Yohimbe has also been used to treat high blood pressure, arteriosclerosis, chest pain, and as a local anesthetic.

Native to West Africa, yohimbe has long been used as an aphrodisiac. Undocumented interactions with psychopharmacological herbs have been reported. Because yohimbe is a short-term MAO inhibitor, it should never be taken with substances that contain the amino acid tyramine. Liver, cheese, red wine, chocolate, beer, aged meats, nuts, and some diet aids and decongestants all include this amino acid.

Dosage: Yohimbe is available with a prescription as the FDA-approved alkaloid yohimbine hydrochloride. (An alkaloid is any of a number of usually pharmacological substances found in plants that combine with acids to make a salt.) It is also available without prescription in extract form, but typical preparations available in health food stores fail to list the dosage, which can lead to dangerous misuse. I personally caution against trying yohimbine without expert advice.

Dosage: Standard dosage is 15 to 20 mg per day, but up to 42 mg per day may prove to be more effective.

Risks: If you have liver or kidney diseases or suffer from mental disorders like schizophrenia, therapeutic yohimbe preparations can be harmful to your health. Possible side effects are anxiety, increased blood pressure, an abnormally fast heart rate, and nausea and vomiting.

Zinc

Zinc works with red blood cells to remove carbon dioxide from the body, helps build bone, and is part of certain enzymes that metabolize protein, carbohydrates, and alcohol. It promotes cell repair and growth, and permits the senses of taste and smell to function normally.

Zinc is an important mineral for male sexual function and the prostate contains the highest concentration of zinc of any body tissue. So if you don't get enough, you may be in danger of prostate problems, low testosterone levels, and low sperm counts.

Zinc inhibits the production of prolactin, a pituitary hormone that can lead to sexual dysfunction. If you do suffer from forms of sexual dysfunction or from BPH, you'll most likely need more than the RDA of zinc. Some evidence suggests that just as a deficiency of the mineral causes sexual problems an abundance of it may help sexual function—even if your problem wasn't originally caused by a zinc deficiency. Studies show that zinc reduces the symptoms of BPH, including prostate enlargement.

Zinc raises testosterone levels and is necessary for hormone metabolism, sperm formation, and sperm motility (it helps the little guys move around). Zinc supplements have thus been shown to effectively aid in fertility.

Zinc is concentrated in semen, and frequent ejaculation can greatly diminish zinc in the body. If a deficiency exists, the body appears to respond by reducing sexual drive as a mechanism by which to hold on to this important trace mineral.

Low zinc levels lead to decreased testosterone levels and sperm counts. It's common to find low zinc levels in infertile men. Although severe zinc deficiency is rare in the United States, marginal deficiency may show up as increased susceptibility to infections, poor wound healing, decreased sense of taste or smell, skin disorders, and impaired sexual function. A study cited in the journal *Nutrition* found that testosterone levels were doubled in a group of men over the age of sixty who took zinc supplements.

Researchers at the Center for the Study of Prostatic Disease at Cook County Hospital studied 5,000 patients with prostate trouble over a 10-year period. They found that zinc appears to prevent prostate enlargement and enhances prostate health overall. And a study performed by Dr. Irving Bush, professor of urology at the University of Chicago, showed that zinc supplements relieved infectious prostatitis in seven out of ten patients treated. In another study conducted at the Department of Urology at First Affiliated Hospital in China researchers looked at the effect that supplementing with organic zinc would have on a group of men suffering from chronic bacterial prostatitis. Men in the study were broken into two groups and both groups were given routine antibiotics but one of the groups was also supplemented with organic zinc. The group that received the zinc supplementation had a measurable improvement in pain, urinary symptoms, quality of life, and maximum urethra closure pressure when compared with the non-zinc group.

Zinc is considered an antioxidant and an anti-aging agent. It is a key component of superoxide dismutase (SOD), an antioxidant the body makes to destroy free radicals that can hasten cell damage and aging. It is an essential component for more than 300 enzyme reactions that support numerous body functions. It is necessary for the body's metabolism of all energy nutrients. Zinc aids in collagen production, giving it a reputation as a wound healer, and serves as a general booster of the immune system (thus aiding in disease prevention).

Modern farming and food processing techniques have resulted in an inadequate supply of zinc in many of the foods we eat. Worse, your body can't effectively store zinc, and therefore needs to replenish its supply regularly.

Researchers hypothesize that zinc may stimulate the thymus, which is related to immune cell development. In a British study at the University of Newcastle, 18 patients whose leg ulcers failed to respond to treatment were found to have lower zinc blood levels than leg-ulcer patients who recovered speedily. After 4 months of zinc therapy, 13 of these 18 nonresponsive patients healed completely. And in an Italian study, researches found that zinc improved certain aspects of the immune function.

Doctors believe zinc deficiency can contribute to cancer of the esophagus by causing it to become inflamed. Symptoms of zinc deficiency can include poor appetite, scaly skin, hair loss, diarrhea, and reduced resistance to infection.

A diet devoid of zinc can delay sexual maturity and even interfere with physical growth. In the 1960s, researchers studied a group of men in the Middle East who were unable to absorb zinc into their systems. "They looked like they were 10 years old when actually they were 20 years old," commented one of the scientists on the research team. "When they got zinc supplements, they actually began to change from boys to men."

United States Department of Agriculture (USDA) biologist Curtis Hunt did a study where zinc intake in 11 men was lowered to 1.4 mg a day—about a tenth of the minimum recommended daily requirement. The result: lower testosterone levels in the blood, and a one-third reduction in semen production.

Dietary zinc can be found in high concentrations in liver, nuts, seeds, oysters, clams, lobster, beef, lamb, crab, turkey, chicken, cereal, beans, cowpeas, egg yolks, fish, milk, oatmeal, potato, peas, soybeans, whole-grain products, wheat germ, sunflower seeds, pumpkin seeds, black-strap molasses, and shitake mushrooms.

Dosage: The recommended daily dosage of zinc citrate supplementation for men seeking to maintain prostate health and sexual potency is 10 mg. Zinc should be taken in a form that is easy for the body to absorb, such as zinc picolinate or zinc citrate. Since copper and zinc compete for absorption in your body, if you take a zinc supplement you should also take a copper supplement to avoid copper deficiency.

The ratio of zinc to copper supplementation should be 7:1 to 14:1. So if you take 10 mg zinc, you should also take, at a different time during the day, about 1 mg copper. Taking vitamin B_6 will further enhance zinc absorption.

The RDA is 12-15 mg. Standard dietary supplements supply 15 mg. It is suggested that if you suffer from erectile dysfunction, low sperm count, chronic prostate infection, or BPH that you eat foods rich in zinc, and that you also take a supplement of 45 mg. Up to 60 mg has been recommended to men suffering from BPH, but this level is significantly higher that the RDA and you of course should consult an expert before taking such high levels of this mineral.

Warning: 150 mg zinc daily has been shown to harm white blood cells and lower the levels of HDL ("good" cholesterol).

To sum up...

- It's not true that all natural supplements are free of side effects—some have them.

- Read the label and follow directions carefully.

- When in doubt, ask your doctor before taking any supplement.

More natural ways to make sex better

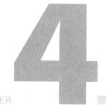

CHAPTER

"Whoever called it necking was a poor judge of anatomy."

—Groucho Marx

Nutrition and nutritional supplements, as we've seen, have the potential to enormously enhance male sexual potency. But they are only part of the picture, and you ignore the foundations of peak sexual performance, including health and self-care, at your peril. By following the tips in this chapter, you can get the maximum benefit out of any supplementation program you follow.

4 steps to achieving better "sexual health"

STEP 1. Regular checkups after 40 or whenever needed.

"Real men don't go to the doctor." A lot of guys think this way. But it's a macho posturing that can ruin your sex life. Worse it could possibly kill you.

Men on average live 7 years less than women. The biggest reasons for the difference, they say, are men drink more than women and visit doctors less frequently than women. Most men see a doctor only when they have a serious complaint. Other factors contributing to our shorter life spans include smoking and hypertension.

Because of the way a man's body works, it makes good sense to start paying regular attention to it after age 40. Even if you are feeling great, an annual prostate exam and a chat with your doctor about blood pressure, weight, diet and exercise makes sense.

While you're at it, get a complete physical. Screening tests can catch many types of cancer early, allowing easier treatment and increasing your longevity. A blood-pressure test can help detect hypertension early enough for it to be treated through diet and exercise, eliminating the need to take blood pressure medication.

If you are experiencing problems with urination or suspect a sexually transmitted disease, don't wait to seek treatment. Your sexual health is based on a healthy body. When it comes to a car, preventive maintenance is a lot cheaper than an engine overhaul. It's the same with your body. And unlike a car, you get only one.

STEP 2. Conduct a stress and health review.

Take a few minutes to think about your overall mental and physical health. If at any point you become concerned about lackluster sexual potency and sex drive, examine recent events in your life. Perhaps they are the cause.

When you're young, "burning the candle at both ends" doesn't seem to have a price. We can get into the habit of pushing our bodies hard and over-riding the warning signs that signal "time for a break." A recent article proclaimed, "Sleep is the Sex of the 2000's." If you fantasize about sleep instead of sex, it's worth noting.

You may identify one or more areas where you need to make some changes... changes that can lead to a much smoother pace of life. Taking time out for a self-review lets you put things in perspective, to ask the question, "Is this right for me?"

During my first marriage, my wife and I were often in conflict. But with my second wife, Eveline, I don't feel in conflict. I occasionally feel that there still might be unresolved issues, but some how they're not so important to me.

I have a theory that most sex tends to die between couples because there is so much unspoken and so much unresolved. Why are you trying to make love with someone, if you really resent her or him, and have been resenting her or him for some time now?

So a big part of taking responsibility is finding ways to keep the air clear between the two of you. And that requires being responsible in communication and in the relationship. You know, the old saying is, women want to make love in order to make up and men want to make up in order to make love. So it's a difficult dance and it is an issue for many, many couples.

Men are particularly vulnerable to certain stress responses at home and work. Today the demands on our time are tremendous. Everyone has too much to do and not enough time to do it. According to an article in one major men's magazine 42 percent of American workers believe they are overloaded with work.

We lose brain matter as we age: Brain weight actually decreases 10 percent between ages 20 and 90. Some researchers believe that men are less able than women to relax their minds when taking breaks from mentally stressing activities. Guys may need physical exercise or nutritional supplements to help alleviate stress.

Just keeping up with the normal events of such a fast-paced society can deter us from wanting to be sexual. What's the solution? Several years ago in a men's workshop, the leader told us, "Make an appointment with your partner." How foolish I thought that was!

Now, I see the wisdom in it. You make an appointment and maybe that seems a little artificial (which it sure did to me when my body was raging with hormones). At the appointed time, you come together. The point is, I see the value in making that appointment, meeting at the prescribed time, putting on some nice music, lighting a candle, you know, maybe some incense, and then just being with your partner as the process unfolds. It's as simple as that.

STEP 3: What's Bugging You?

A satisfying sex life is partly an expression of a satisfying life. Rather than focus on what's not happening sexually, sometimes it's worth stopping for a minute and looking at other aspects of your life. Our culture has a tendency to emphasize sex as a way to solve problems rather than an expression of happiness.

Good sex is a result of balanced living, not a solution to a problem. If your sex life has to make up for things not going right elsewhere, it's carrying a very heavy load. Sometimes the chance to talk things out with a friend or professional counselor is all that's required. Even the most stable relationships go through ups and downs, and your partner may suggest marriage counseling or group therapy at some point.

In my own sex life with my partner, I think about trying to focus on what's happening at the moment, and not let my mind wander. When we're lying in bed together I try to be aware of how our intimacy and physical closeness feels physically and mentally. I'm exploring this one moment after another. And if I am functioning optimally, what I tell myself is: you don't have to know where this is going, but you do have to require yourself to stay in the present.

It's really about just sharing the day, sharing the moment, in a soft way: being together without having an agenda, not "This is really going to have to go some place." It isn't so much about stimulation or about arousal, it is more about being together. If arousal happens in the process, that's nice. If it doesn't happen, that's fine.

A partnership that is incompatible is not the basis for a happy sex life. And one that needs better communication can't be fixed by sex.

Many therapists believe that anger and resentment can lead to impotence. Let's face it. It's pretty obvious that when you are angry it is difficult to enjoy sex and even more difficult to help your partner enjoy it. Impotence can result as a symptom of repressed anger. Some experts theorize that in some cases impotence can even be an unconscious way to vent your anger by depriving your partner of pleasure or satisfaction while avoiding responsibility for your angry feelings.

Seeking help isn't failure. It's a rational decision to make things better. And the rewards—including greater sexual satisfaction—can be substantial.

STEP 4: Have reasonable expectations.

Be realistic in your erotic expectations as well as all other aspects of your life. "Happy the man who early learns the wide chasm that lies between his wishes and his powers," said Johann von Goethe.

Each person has a different sexual "personality." Their appetite and interest in sex may be different from other people from the very beginning. In fact, a recent extensive survey of American sexual behavior indicated that people were having less sex, more conventional sex, and more satisfying sex than the experts had proclaimed over the last twenty years.

By and large, people work out their sex lives for themselves by themselves. It's wrapped up in love, family, work and community. It's not separated out into a "task" or "exercise." A good sex life is one that works for you and your partner. It will involve compromise; it always does. And it can often go through periods of greater or lesser physical expression.

Many couples go through periods of celibacy without stress. A new baby is a classic reason for a "dry spell." Yet we also know that close to 30 percent of the male population has few or no sexual experiences during any given year. So depending on where we live and with whom we live, our experiences are considered "normal" or not.

Quickie Quiz

Answer true or false to the following six statements.

❶ I feel confident that I can get and maintain an erection that is hard enough to enter my partner.

❷ My overall desire for sex is moderate to high

❸ When I have sexual intercourse I always maintain an erection until satisfactory completion

❹ As a general rule I rarely worry about successful sexual performance

❺ Overall I would rate my sex life as moderately to very satisfying

❻ When I attempt to have sex it is almost always a satisfactory experience for me.

If you answered false to two or more of the above statements you might want to consider talking to a professional about erectile dysfunction.

The bottom line is that there is no reason why your sex life needs to match up with everyone else's. You don't drive the same car, watch the same TV programs or subscribe to the same magazines. While statistics are interesting you're not ever going to be able to live someone else's sex life. And why should you?

Roadblocks to Sexual Contentment

The vicious cycle of sexual unhappiness has been experienced by many men. Expectations about performance are frustrated. That leads to anxiety or self-consciousness. The anxiety leads to more expectations being frustrated. And so on. If we were teaching a kid to hit a baseball, we'd recognize the problem quickly. In ourselves, it's tougher to spot, tougher to correct.

Removing these roadblocks to contentment means recognizing that the entire negative cycle will rebuild itself given a chance. So we have to moderate our expectations and control our anxiety, roughly at the same time. Ignorance, poor health, and unrealistic expectations form a trio that sabotage many men's happiness.

The first step? Changing the situation in any number of ways is going to have a positive effect, whether it's easing up on coffee or getting an extra hour's sleep. Perhaps we just need to get away with our significant other for a relaxed weekend in the country. Or maybe we require something more intensive, such as a weekend seminar with our partner to revisit what it is we actually like about marriage or partnership. Or it may be something more profound. Perhaps our physical health is compromising our sexual abilities and we need a checkup. Whatever it is, taking a concrete step is going to increase our confidence and reduce our anxiety.

Part of setting realistic expectations is learning to live with what we cannot change. There is no doubt that serious injury or disease will affect our sexual experience and our means of expressing sexuality.

Similarly, if we hold onto a teenager's view of sex while trying to perform in the present, we are almost sure to be disappointed. Don't let Hollywood, or the boy you were at 16, dictate how you live your life today.

Your sexual appetite and enjoyment with a long-term partner is always going to be different than with a casual relationship. For some men, that difference is unbearable. For others, it's what makes it worthwhile. Either way, finding a balance between your abilities and expectations will keep sex from seeming as frenetic an exercise as a pet hamster running on a treadmill.

When we recognize the vicious cycle, and fully recognize that things we cannot change, then what's left? Basically life. Life's going to dish up a series of surprises. It's also going to change constantly. Things are going to go well for you and not for your partner, then the next week, the reverse. Keeping a sense of humor and a sense of perspective will keep you content, in your sex life and in life as a whole.

In my opinion prescription ED drugs are often an attempt to go back to the past, rather than to be willing to explore what is right here, right now and work with what is right now. The natural alternatives described in chapters 3 can help you get and maintain a stiff erection, but they also build mood, desire, energy, and pleasure. A prescription drug however is purely a "boner pill"—it gives you the wood, so to speak, but not the will.

A prescription-induced session in the bedroom can become an attempt to recapture youth rather than being comfortable with the limitations and the richness of maturity. There are so many possibilities in having an experience with someone you've known for a long time, yourself, and in some cases, your mate, because there's a lot of possibility in the mutually shared experience of a lasting relationship.

Male sexual health isn't mysterious. Our culture, which emphasizes an Olympic ideal of sex as competitive sport, really works against us. Maintaining lifelong sexual satisfaction is a matter of adapting to change and giving our body the best possible foundation for sexuality.

Good Health, Good Sex

Good sexual health is based on our overall health. Proper diet, exercise, rest and recreation are essential to give the body the energy and state of relaxation necessary for deeply satisfying sex. One's mental attitude is also strengthened by good physical health. A small change in our behavior can lead to large benefits in sexual health.

The prostate, which is a focal point of our urinary and reproductive tracts, is subject to a number of irritating ailments. As we age, it can be the cause of problems. Taking care of those problems and adapting our lifestyle can mean a much more satisfying sex life.

If we want to enhance our sexual health, we can also look to exercises and nutrition that increase our vitality and provide essential nutrients to those organs associated with sexuality. A growing number of nutrients are available to us in supplements and special foods. They are a proven way to make a change in our sexual health. If sex has become an athletic event in our lives, then why not train and eat like an athlete?

There's nothing unique about sexual health and happiness. Common sense goes a long way. Identify the things you can correct, accept the things that can't be changed, and realize that it's your sex life, not someone else's. In the ups and downs of a sexual relationship, your long-term contentment is what counts.

DID YOU KNOW?

Heavy smoking can lead to damage of the tiny blood vessels in the penis.

The Fitter the Better: Improved Fitness Means Improved Sexual Vitality

Overall body conditioning includes a wide range of basic health indicators, which are all too familiar. Our weight should be within a normal range for our age and build. Our diet should include a proper mix of proteins and starches. Fruits, vegetables, and whole grains should be a part of everyone's diet. The direct bene-fits of exercise for the cardiac system, for stress reduction, and better sexual activi-ty, even for previously sedentary and healthy middle-aged men, are well docu-mented...but widely ignored.

STUDY RESULTS

According to a long term study published in the journal Archives of Internal Medicine the latest research shows that regular exercise reduces older men's risk of developing prostate cancer. In fact it was found that for men over 65 that engaged in at least three hours physical activity per week such as biking or swimming had a 70% lower risk of being diagnosed with the cancer or dying from the disease.

Arch Intern Med. 2005 May 9;165(9):1005-10.

A prospective study of physical activity and incident and fatal prostate cancer.

Giovannucci EL, Liu Y, Leitzmann MF, Stampfer MJ, Willett WC.
Department of Nutrition, Harvard School of Public Health, Boston, Mass, USA.

BACKGROUND: Whether physical activity has benefits against prostate cancer incidence or progression is unclear. Therefore, we assessed physical activity in relation to prostate cancer incidence, mortality, and Gleason histologic grade.

METHODS: We used data from the Health Professionals Follow-up Study, a prospective cohort study, to determine the number of cases of incident, advanced (seminal vesicle invasion, metastasis, or fatal), fatal, and high-grade prostate cancer in a cohort of 47,620 US male health professionals, followed up from February 1, 1986, to January 31, 2000.

RESULTS: During 14 years of follow-up, we documented 2892 new cases of prostate cancer, including 482 advanced cases (280 of which were fatal). For total prostate cancer, no association was observed for total, vigorous, and nonvigorous physical activity. In men 65 years or older, we observed a lower risk in the highest category of vigorous activity for advanced (multivariable relative risk, 0.33; 95% confidence interval, 0.17-0.62, for more than 29 vs 0 metabolic equivalent hours) and for fatal (relative risk, 0.26; 95% confidence interval, 0.11-0.66) prostate cancer. No associations were observed in younger men. Differential screening by prostate-specific antigen or a reduction in physical activity due to undiagnosed prostate cancer did not appear to account for the results. Among cases, men with high levels of physical activity were less likely to be diagnosed with poorly differentiated cancers (Gleason grade > or = 7).

CONCLUSION: Although the mechanisms are not yet understood, these findings suggest that regular vigorous activity could slow the progression of prostate cancer and might be recommended to reduce mortality from prostate cancer, particularly given the many other documented benefits of exercise.

PMID: 15883238
[PubMed - indexed for MEDLINE]

Sexuality as we age does not have to be the slippery slope to sexual inadequacy as is commonly assumed. The climb to peaks of sexual pleasure will become and remain easier if you observe some basic physical and dietary needs still required by your maturing body.

We've all heard regular exercise is important, but will it really improve a man's sex life? The answer to this question is a resounding "YES!" It's been studied, documented and shown that the benefits of consistent exercise include a reduction in heart disease risk factors and increase in overall fitness. But there are other major documented benefits to fitness including increased frequency of various intimate activities, greater reliability of more-than-adequate functioning during sex, and a higher percentage of satisfying orgasms.

The first thing to do in starting an exercise program is to turn off the TV and get off the couch. Next is to make sure you are fit enough. If you have been mostly inactive for a number of years or have been previously diagnosed with an illness, start slowly and consult your physician—and perhaps a personal trainer—first. If you find you are fit enough to begin, the next thing is to select an activity that you feel you would enjoy.

Recharging your sex drive may be a simple as taking a walk with your partner, with or without the dog, before you go to sleep. Or, maybe it's time to jump on that long avoided exercise bike or treadmill for a gentle workout. Not only will you sleep more soundly but a healthy routine can also increase your desire for sex, improve your performance, your satisfaction and your partner's. It's not necessary to approach sex as an athletic event to be timed, judged, and reviewed. Nevertheless, it is a physical activity and, as with any physical challenge, you can prepare your body.

> **TIPS**
>
> Remember that sexual function naturally changes with age. As we get older adding a little more stimulation and allowing for a longer period of time to achieve an erection are good ideas. And trust me you are not going to hear any complaints from your partner about taking a little extra time!

To keep your sex life from shriveling, don't let your body shrivel! Some form of full-body exercise, even gentle, is necessary to improve not only your physical ability but to improve your sexual desire and orgasms. The best exercises are the kind that get your heart moving. Fast walking, swimming, bicycling, and cross-country skiing are excellent ways of maintaining physical health—as long as you don't overdo it.

Building Sexual Muscle

While aerobic and endurance types of exercises play their part in keeping us healthy, regular sex or self-pleasuring is as important, if not more so. Directly exercising the muscles related to sexual activity and release is another worthwhile activity, commonly overlooked. Your abdomen, hips, buttocks and thighs are the important large muscles to keep active, but especially important are the smaller muscles around the anus and at the base of the scrotum. If we take a tip from the wisdom of other cultures, western men would do well to exercise these internal muscles related to sexual activity.

If you ever have been forced to stay in bed, been immobile, or worn a cast for an extended period of time, you probably know how your muscles shrink, atrophy, and become weakened when not used. This is equally true of your sex muscles: the PC and the anal sphincter. Two or three inches of your penis (see Figure. 1 in Chapter 1 on page 14) is rooted inside the body in a muscle known as the "PC" or pubococcygeus (pronounced PEW-bo-cox-si-gee-us), and this muscle can be felt, exercised, and developed.

Since the penis itself is made up primarily of spongy tissue and contains no muscle fibers, you can't enlarge it, like your biceps, with exercise. But you can maintain its "support system" and gain more control over its emissions. Strengthening these muscles will enhance your staying power and the intensity of sensations during sex.

The penis actually withdraws into the body if it is not regularly used, as many men who are not sexually active have witnessed. Fortunately, we know the penis can be turned around and brought back to the playing field for the next round of games.

While many men may think about the anus as something "dirty" or "unnatural" to stimulate, its proximity to the prostate and its own high concentration of nerve endings make the anus a highly sensitive, erogenous zone, as many men—both gay and straight—have discovered. If you do experiment with direct, pleasurable stimulation of the lowest, inside muscles in your anus, you should remember to make sure everything is super clean before you do and make sure to wash up thoroughly before touching your partner.

Just like the PC, we can exercise the ring-like sphincter muscle that contracts the anus, in order to gain some control over the progression of events that occur almost involuntarily as your body sensations escalate during orgasm. In order to make sex more scintillating, we would be wise to make orgasms sequence more "voluntary."

The following exercises, drawn from ancient Chinese practices, can help develop your sexual energy and sensitivity:

- Belly Breathing
- Stopping the Stream
- The PC Pull-Up.

Belly Breathing

Strange as it may seem, strengthening and deepening your breathing is the first step toward learning to control your ejaculation and to handle greater sensation in your lovemaking body. As a side benefit it will also enhance your ability to listen to your partner, appreciate her in trying moments, and to take feedback from her. Most of us breathe very shallowly, generally into our chest and shoulders. This allows only a small amount of oxygen to be absorbed by our lungs.

Belly breathing—breathing deeply into the bottom of your lungs and into your diaphragm—is

Belly Breathing Exercise

The following simple exercise illustrates the shallow chest breathing typical in the Western world while helping you to concentrate on proper belly breathing. Proper breathing can have a powerful effect on your energy levels and health.

1. Lie down in a comfortable place with your knees bent and your feet flat on the floor or bed. Place your hand on your tummy and simply observe your breathing and the movement of your hand. Do not try to change your normal breathing pattern. Most likely you will notice that your belly hardly moves, only your chest, and your tummy may even move inwards slightly. This shallow breathing pattern is typical in the Western world.

2. Now on your next breathe concentrate on breathing deeply into your belly and allowing it to expand outward as you take in air. As you breathe out allow your belly to retract. There is no need to force these movements, just be mindful of the breathing and movement. If you find this at all difficult, of if your belly seems to tight, you can very gently press on your tummy as you exhale and then as you inhale gradually release this tension.

3. Continue to take these deep belly breathes for several minutes. When you feel ready to stop, take a moment to be aware of how the deep breathing made you feel. Many people report feeling more relaxed and energized. Your body is probably not used to getting the proper amounts of oxygen and you might experience some lightheadedness the first couple of times you do this exercise so be sure to get up slowly.

the way newborn children and professional singers breathe. This is the healthiest way to breathe, but we lose this natural ability as stress and anxiety cause us to cut our breathing short.

The first step is to become conscious of or breathing. Whenever you take a breath try to inhale and exhale through your nose. This filters and warms the air. Our noses are not just a sense organ and an opening for air; they also condition and moisten the air as it enters the body. When you inhale through your mouth, it is harder for the body to assimilate and use the air.

Next add in a few minutes of belly breathing each day. This will teach your body to breathe more deeply on its own, even while you sleep. Although it is not as important to exhale through your nose as it is to inhale, it is still preferable. If you find it easier to exhale through the mouth when breathing deeply, that's fine. Just see what works best for you.

If you are having a hard time with belly breathing, you might try belly laughing instead. A belly laugh is the kind that makes your whole abdomen shake and somewhat ache. Since we're not used to contracting these muscles very often, the exercise helps tone them considerably.

Stopping the Stream

Now it's time to develop your sexual strength. The PC is a muscular sling that stretches from the pubic bone in front to the tailbone at the back tip of your butt. This is the muscle you use to stop yourself from urinating when you can't find a toilet, or to push out those last few drops of urine. As mentioned earlier, the PC is also responsible for the rhythmic contractions in your pelvis and anus during orgasm.

Your orgasm builds from your prostate, so learning how to squeeze on the prostate with your pelvic muscles is essential. In addition to having more and better orgasms, this exercise can help prevent hardening and swelling of the prostate as well as other prostate problems.

The PC muscle is also the one that allows animals to wag their tails. In fact, the word penis literally means "tail" in Latin. So what you are going to do with these exercises is learn to "wag your tail" to strengthen your erections and intensify your orgasms.

An easy way to find and feel your PC muscles is to stop the flow of urine by clamping down inside your groin the next time you urinate. Stopping yourself from peeing was one of the first acts of control you learned to have over your body. Using your ability to control your urine flow can now help you control and strengthen your ejaculation.

The most important part of this exercise is to stop and start urinating as many times as you can. One man describes his "peeing practice" this way: "Whenever I go to the bathroom now, I try to stop and go at least three times. And if I'm in a fun mood and I am not in a rush, I will try to just stop, go, stop, go, sometimes five or six or seven times."

The PC Pull-Ups

The importance of the PC muscle was discovered in the West during the 1940's by Arnold Kegel, a gynecologist. He developed the famous Kegel exercise, which allows pregnant women to gain control over their bladders and uterine muscles, to ease the ordeal of childbirth. Strengthening this muscle is equally important for a man's pelvic health and sexual pleasure.

The muscles around the eyes, mouth, prostate, and anus are all what are known anatomically as "circular" muscles in the body. In eastern thought and sexual medicine it is believed that they are all connected, so that by squeezing the muscles around your eyes and mouth, you can increase the force of your PC Pull-Ups. You might look a little silly but I'd say it's certainly worth a try.

TIPS

Both men and women have a PC (pubococcygeus) muscle, which lines the pelvic floor. Exercising this muscle and keeping it in shape can pay off in the bedroom in helping you to achieve stronger and longer lasting erections.

To locate your PC muscle the next time you urinate stop the flow midstream .The muscle you used to do this is the one we want to target. Now that you know where your PC muscle is you should start exercising it every day.

You can do the exercises just about anywhere. At least once a day try the following exercise: Tighten your PC muscle and hold for a count of 5, and release. Repeat 10 times. Try to keep all the surrounding muscles relaxed while you do this.

The most important thing is to practice contracting and releasing your PC muscle, as often as you can. You can do your PC exercises while driving, while watching TV, while sending a fax, or while attending a meeting. See how many contractions you can do while waiting at a red light, or hold a single contraction until the light turns green!

You Are What You Eat

While changes are part and parcel of our species' aging process, there are factors that can enhance a maturing man's vintage sexual prowess. Proper diet, rest, exercise, and attitude can help to keep the fire of sexual energy burning bright.

Anything that unduly stresses the body is going to have an impact on sexual health. Your overall diet and attitude toward your body's health is going to influence things markedly. Some environmental influences can be overcome by examining and altering lifestyle, and some by adding certain necessary vitamins and minerals to rebuild and strengthen your inner biological terrain.

Despite the fact that more than 70% of the American public consumes some form of vitamin and mineral supplementation, mainstream medicine has been slow to recommend vitamins unless an actual clinical deficiency is identified. It is wise to consider consulting a nutritional counselor in addition to an open-minded MD or a naturopathic doctor in order to plot a regimen that suits your individual body and health history.

Chapter 3 reviewed nutrients that have a good track record in

What's for Dinner? Serving Up Aphrodisiac Fun

An aphrodisiac is any substance that arouses sexual desire. The word aphrodisiac is of Green origin meaning sexual pleasures and is derived from the name of the Greek goddess of love Aphrodite. Records of aphrodisiac foods abound throughout history ranging from Chinese Masters to ancient Greeks.

Although there has never been total agreement on which foods are aphrodisiac in nature a number of them have appeared over and over again in literature throughout the ages. Many of these were foods that by nature represented seed or semen such as bulbs or eggs, others found there way onto the list because of their physical resemblance to male or female genitalia, and still others have more mysterious origins.

Following is a list of some foods commonly thought to have aphrodisiac qualities. Why not test the theory and serve some up tonight?

- Peaches
- Bananas
- Avocados
- Asparagus
- Basil
- Almonds
- Cucumbers
- Onions
- Arugula
- Pine Nuts
- Caviar
- Aniseed
- Mussels
- Oysters
- Chocolate
- Figs
- Radish
- Truffles
- Artichokes

supporting male health while indirectly but substantially improving your sexual fire. You can discuss these with your health care practitioner or read more about them on your own (see the appendixes for additional helpful information). Keep in mind that a healthy diet and exercise are the foundation of any supplement plan. However, if you notice unusual changes in how your body is behaving or operating, or suspect any of the conditions mentioned above, professional medical advice is advised.

Love Potion Number Nine

Herbal aphrodisiacs have been the target of investigation for thousands of years. Do they exist?

Literature from a variety of cultures is full of references to aphrodisiacs, which reportedly worked for some people some of the time. Most of these substances appear to work by promoting good overall health, including reproductive system health, and thereby enhancing sexual vitality. Herbalists recommend herbs like ginkgo to improve circulation and mental acuity; saw palmetto to nourish the prostate and retard BPH; the Chinese herb astragalus to stimulate sperm production; bee pollen and royal jelly to tone the genito-urinary tract and prevent ailments (see Chapter 3.)

The Chinese have a history of identifying successful aphrodisiacs and herbs that can strengthen the male sexual organs. One of the most well known herbal families includes the ginsengs, which have had a long history as aphrodisiacs as well as having overall health benefits. They contain a rich supply of steroid-like compounds.

Panax and Siberian ginsengs are known as adaptogens. Adaptogens strengthen the body and have a normalizing effect against disease. Like a thermostat maintaining a constant temperature in a house, adaptogenic ginsengs work via the nervous system to smooth out the responses to various kinds of inner and outer stressors.

There are several herbs that relate directly to the biochemistry of erection. Damiana has a long tradition in America as a sexual stimulant. Potency wood, also known as muira puama, is from a South American plant and has been recently investigated as an aphrodisiac and nerve stimulant for erection problems.

Pygeum africanum is from an African evergreen tree whose bark has traditionally been used to treat urinary tract disorders and to enhance the function of the prostate gland, its primary target organ in men. Yohimbe bark, from a tree native to West Africa, acts to increase libido as well as blood flow to erectile tissue. These herbs have recently received a resurgence of interest by those formulating combinations to enhance male sexual vigor. But yohimbe has perhaps more warnings and side effects than any other male potency supplements made from plants; be sure to read the description in chapter 3 carefully and consult your physician before deciding whether to take it.

A Body Affair

Sex is a whole-body affair. Your ability to cultivate and circulate your sexual energy only increases with more practice and experience. Your sexuality will no doubt change over time, and you may miss some of the feeding frenzy of youth. But the more refined pleasures of older age can be just as delectable as youthful folly, if not more so.

Good health should not just be thought of as the absence of disease. Health results from supplying what is essential to your body on a daily basis, while disease comes when you deny these essentials and try to live without giving your body what it needs. At one time we all thought that we were invincible: that no matter how we ate, drank, smoked or pushed ourselves, we would somehow stay healthy, full of energy, and sexually strong forever. But all that changes as you approach and hit 40. You begin to realize that you are mortal.

The last few decades of research and the rise of heart disease, cancers, and other illnesses have told us that the body has its limits. We can abuse our health, ignore it, and put Band-Aids on signs that show we are wearing down our essential reserves. Or, we can pay attention more to our bodies, take charge of our diet and the stress we subject ourselves to, so that our health will support and sustain us for years to come. The choice is yours. I pray you choose wisely.

To sum up…

- If you are experiencing erectile dysfunction, have a checkup. The causes are sometimes physical problems that can be corrected with proper medical treatment.

- Practice the exercises in this chapter (belly breathing, stream stopping, PC pull-ups). They can increase your performance and satisfaction.

- Don't put yourself or your spouse under the pressure of having to have great intercourse (or even any intercourse) every time. Start with affection, communication, cuddling, and snuggling. Let things build naturally and see what happens.

- Remember the old saying, "It's not what happens to you in life; it's how you handle it." As we get older, we encounter all kinds of problems—mental, physical, and emotional—we could not have ever imagined in our youth. But when it comes to regaining intimacy and pleasure in the bedroom, there are positive steps you can take to reawaken your sex life again. Whether sex dies or lives in your life is largely under your control. My advice? Natural alternatives to prescription drugs work! Try them until you find the one that works for you.

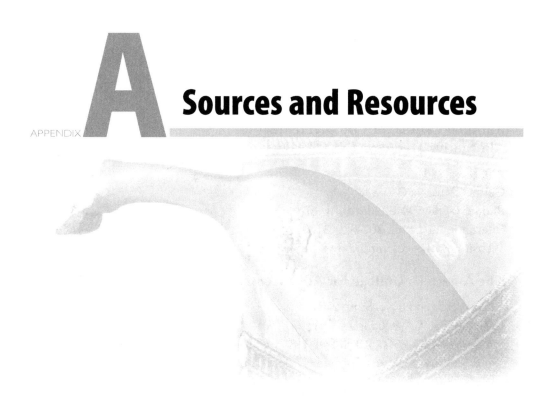

APPENDIX

A Sources and Resources

Organizations

Impotents Anonymous

2020 Pennsylvania Avenue NW, Suite 929
Washington, DC 20006
Phone: 410-715-9605

Impotence Information Center

PO Box 9
Minneapolis, MN 55440
Phone: 1-800-843-4315

Sexual Function Health Council
American Foundation for Urological Disease

1000 Corporate Boulevard, Suite 410
Linthicum, Maryland 21090
Phone: 1-800-242-2383 or 410-689-3990
Website: www.afud.org
Website: www.impotence.org

National Center for Complementary and Alternative Medicine (NCCAM)

P.O. Box 7923
Gaithersburg, MD 20898
Phone: 1-888-644-6226 (toll-free)
International/Local: 301-519-3153
Website: www.nccam.nih.gov

The American College for Advancement in Medicine (ACAM)

23121 Verdugo Drive, Suite 204
Laguna Hills, CA 92653
Phone: 949-583-7666 or toll free 1-800-532-3688
Website: www.acam.org (provides referrals to naturopathic physicians)

American Association for Naturopathic Physicians (AANP)

3201 New Mexico Ave., N.W. Suite 350
Washington, DC 20016
Phone: 202-895-1392 or toll free 1-866-538-2267
Website: www.naturopathic.org

American Botanical Council

6200 Manor Rd, Austin, TX 78723
Phone: 512-926-4900
Website: www.herbalgram.org

Nutritional Supplements Manufacturers and Distributors

Puritan's Pride

Phone: 1-800-645-1030
Website: www.puritanspride.com

GNC
General Nutrition

888-462-2548
Phone: 1-800-477-4462
Website: www.gnc.com

Life Extension Foundation

PO Box 229120
Hollywood, FL 33022
Phone: 1-800-544-4440
Website: www.lef.org

Vitamin Express

1400 Shattuck Avenue
Berkeley, CA 94709
Phone: 1-800-500-0733
International callers: +1-415-564-8160
Website: www.vitaminexpress.com

The Vitamin Shoppe

2101 91st Street
North Bergen, NJ 07047
Phone: 1-800-223-1216
Website: www.vitaminshoppe.com

Drugstore.com

Phone: 1-800-378-4786
Website: www.drugstore.com

Discreet Adult Shopping

Tootimid – vacuum erection devices, penis rings, adult toys

21 B Olympia Avenue
Woburn, Massachusetts 01801
Phone: 1-888-660-8970
Fax: 781-933-9635
Website: www.tootimid.com

Good Vibrations – penis pumps, penis rings, adult toys

938 Howard Street, Suite 101
San Francisco, CA 94103
Phone: 1-800-289-8423 or 415-974-8990
Fax: 415-974-8989
Website: www.goodvibes.com

Sex Toy Shoppers – penis pumps, rings, adult toys

RPT Ventures, Inc.
1204 NE 8th Street
Gresham, OR. 97030
Website: www.sextoyshoppers.com

Glossary

Alkaloid—a nitrogen-based substance found in plants.

Amino acid—organic compounds from which proteins are synthesized.

Andropause—male menopause.

Antioxidant—a substance that prevents deterioration caused by oxidation.

Aphrodisiac—any substance that awakens sexual desire.

Arteriosclerosis—hardening of the arteries.

Atherosclerosisa—common type of arteriosclerosis.

ATP (adenosine triphosphate)—an enzyme aiding protein reactions that help muscles perform.

Ayurvedic—ancient India medical and healing practice.

BPH (benign prostate hyperplasia)—nonmalignant enlargement of the prostate.

BPH Stage I—symptoms include increase in frequency of urination, pollakiuria, nocturea, delayed onset of urination, weak urinary stream.

BPH Stage II—symptoms include decompensation of the bladder function, formation of residual urine, and urge to urinate.

Chelation—a chemical process through which metals and other substances are removed from the body.

Coenzyme—a substance that binds with protein to form an active enzyme.

Collagen—the fibrous material of which bone, cartilage, and connective tissue are made.

Decoction—substance prepared by boiling.

Dihydrotesterone—formed from testosterone. Too much dihydrotesterone in older men may contribute to enlargement of the prostate.

Diuretic—a substance that causes you to urinate.

Dyseria—painful or difficult urination.

Endocrine—ductless glands whose secretions pass directly from the cells of the gland into the bloodstream.

Enzyme—a protein molecule that causes chemical reactions of other substances without being changed in the process.

Erectile dysfunction—any problems relating to achieving or sustaining an erection.

FDA—Food and Drug Administration.

Flavonoids—compounds found in plants, especially those with yellow and red pigmentation.

Free radicals—a chemically reactive atom or group of atoms having at least one unpaired electron.

Gonads—in men, the testicles; in women, the ovaries.

HDL (high-density lipoprotein)—good cholesterol.

Hemoglobin—a protein in which oxygen is transported through the bloodstream.

Herb—a plant with a fleshy (rather than wooden) stem.

Hormone—a substance made in one organ and conveyed, via the bloodstream, to another organ whose function it stimulates by means of chemical activity.

Hypoglycemic—having low levels of glucose in the bloodstream.

Hypothyroidism—having an underactive thyroid.

Impotence—inability to achieve an erection.

Infusion—liquid made by steeping a substance in water.

LDL (low-density lipoproteins)—bad cholesterol.

Legume—a pea or bean with a pod containing seeds.

Micromole—unit of measure used by scientists to denote a small quantity.

Mineral—naturally occurring inorganic substance with a crystalline structure.

Mitochondria—the part of a cell that converts food to energy.

Neurotransmitter—substances that transmit nerve signals between the nerves.

Nocturea—excessive urination at night.

Nucleic acids—refers to RNA and DNA.

Pubococcygeus—muscle found at the base of the penis.

Pheromone—a substance released by your body that can be detected by other individuals, causing certain reactions in them, including sexual attraction to the person secreting the pheromone.

Pollakiuria—abnormal frequent urination.

Polysaccharide—a complex carbohydrate made up of different sugar molecules.

Precursor—a thing that precedes and indicates something to come.

Prostate cancer, early stage—cancer confined to the prostate.

Prostate cancer, late stage—cancer that has spread beyond the prostate.

Provitamin—substance from which your body can make a vitamin.

RDA—FDA's recommended daily dosage of a vitamin or other supplement.

Reich, Wilhelm—Austrian doctor and psychotherapist.

Semen—seed of a plant or sperm of a male animal.

Spermatorrhea—excessive and involuntary ejaculation without copulation.

Steroid—a substance that supports and bolsters the hormone system.

Superoxide dismutase (SOD)—an important antioxidant that helps fight free radicals capable of causing cellular damage.

Synovial—a lubricating fluid contained in joints and tendons.

Tantric—relating to Hindu or Buddhist mysticism and philosophy.

Tincture—a component of a substance extracted by means of a solvent.

Thermogenic—a substance producing heat.

Triglycerides—a fat made from carbohydrates.

Varicoceles—blocked veins in the groin region similar to varicose veins in the legs.

Vitamins—naturally occurring substances in plants and animals essential for controlling metabolic processes.

Voiding—excessive daytime urination.

APPENDIX C **Index**

Note: Page numbers in **bold** indicate the main discussion of a topic.
Page numbers followed by letters *f* and *t* refer to figures and tables, respectively.

About the Authors

JOHN BYINGTON

JOHN BYINGTON, for many years was CEO and Director of Southwest Research Institute, a New Mexico-based R&D facility researching natural alternatives to pharmaceuticals for treating male potency. After suffering from colon cancer and prostate cancer in his 40s, John became severely "sexually challenged." He credits taking nutritional supplements for restoring him to full male potency and an active sex life.

John is a graduate of the Law School at the University of Nebraska. He lived a conventional middle-class life until about age 40. He then divorced, and at the same time embarked on a series of entrepreneurial ventures in the Midwest and California.

"About half a dozen years ago, I met and married my second wife, Eveline, a free-spirited and spiritually oriented European woman who led me into a life of which I'd had no previous inkling," says John. "We participated in a number of enlightening workshops including Eastern Tantra, emotional release work, and transpersonal psychology. Of course, I was confronted in ways I had never been before."

About the Authors

ROBERT W. BLY

ROBERT W. BLY is a freelance writer and the author of more than forty-five books, including *The Ultimate Unauthorized Stephen King Trivia Challenge* (Kensington), *Start and Run a Successful Mail Order Business* (Self Counsel Press), and *101 Ways to Make Every Second Count* (Career Press). Bob's articles have appeared in such publications as *Cosmopolitan, Amtrak Express, New Jersey Monthly*, and *Writer's Digest.* He has appeared on dozens of radio and TV shows including CBS' "Hard Copy" and CNBC, and has been featured in national media ranging from *Nation's Business* to *The National Inquirer.* Bob is a member of the American Foundation for Urologic Disease.